Praise for Jonathan Research and Program

"I am often asked when there will be a proven prescription for weight loss. This is that prescription."
- **Harvard Medical School's** Dr. Theodoros Kelesidis

"A treasure trove of reliable information...hot, hot hot!"
- **Harvard Medical School's** Dr. JoAnne Manson

"Reveals the real story of diet, exercise, and their effects on us. I heartily recommend this." - **Harvard Medical School's** Dr. John J. Ratey

"Opens the black box of fat loss and makes it simple!"
- **Dr. Oz's Personal Trainer** Joel Harper

"I'm a big fan" - **World's Top Trainer and Creator of P90X** Tony Horton

"Will do more to assist people with their health than all the diet books out there put together. I want to shout, 'Bravo! Finally someone gets it!'"
- Dr. Christiane Northrup, **New York Times best-selling author** of *Women's Bodies, Women's Wisdom* and *The Wisdom of Menopause*

"Provides a powerful set of tools for creating lifelong health!"
- Dr. Mark Hyman, **New York Times best-selling author** of *The Blood Sugar Solution* and *The Daniel Plan*

"An easily understood and applied framework that will change the way you live, look, and feel... will end your confusion once and for all."
- Dr. William Davis, **New York Times best-selling author** of *Wheat Belly*

"Cuts through the noise around weight loss and tells it to us straight."
- Dr. Sara Gottfried, **New York Times best-selling author** of *The Hormone Cure* and *The Hormone Reset Diet*

"Readers will find that focusing on the kinds of foods they are eating can boost their brain power and help them lose the extra ten pounds."
- Dr. Daniel G. Amen, **New York Times best-selling author** of *Change Your Brain, Change Your Body*

"Will change the way you look at dieting!"
- JJ Virgn, **New York Times best-selling author** of *The Virgin Diet*

See hundreds more medical reviews and success stories at:
www.SANESolution.com

To my best friend, partner, and wife, Angela. Just the thought of you brings me more joy, more satisfaction, and more life than anything else I have ever experienced. You are my beloved, without reservation or qualification, as we dance into eternity.

To my heroes and parents, Mary Rose and Robert. All that I am is thanks to your love, example, and support. From the day I was born, and every day after, you have always found a way to help and love me. I live, hoping to return the favor.

To my friends and partners, Scott, Tyler, Sean, Abhishek, April, Lori, Wednesday, Josh, Jason, Andrea, and Rebecca, my delightful sister Patty, my wonderful brothers Tim, Cameron, and Branden, and my loving in-laws Terry and Carolyn. You are such treasures. Thank you for being who you are and thank you for meaning so much to me.

To you and the hundreds of thousands of other SANE family members all around the world with the courage to eat and exercise smarter. You have taken the road less traveled and it will make all the difference.

Published in the Worldwide by Yopti, LLC (SANESolution) New York. Seattle. California. www.SANESolution.com.

None of work may be reproduced, stored, or distributed in any form or by any means except as permitted under Section 107 or 108 of the 1976 United States Copyright Act, without first obtaining written permission of the Publisher, or authorization through payment of the appropriate per-copy fee to the Copyright Clearance Center, 222 Rosewood Drive, Danvers, MA, 01923, (978) 750-8400, or on the web at www.copyright.com. Requests to the Publisher for permission should be sent to SANESolution.com/contact.

SANE books can be purchased at quantity discounts to use as premiums, promotions, or for corporate training programs. For more information on bulk pricing please email Yopti, LLC at SANESolution.com/contact.

Editor: Mary Rose Bailor
Production: Abhishek Pandey
Exterior Design: Tyler Archer

Publisher's Cataloging-in-Publication
Bailor, Jonathan.
99 Calorie Myth and SANE Certified Main Dish Recipes Volume 1: Lose Weight, Increase Energy, Improve Your Mood, Fix Digestion, and Sleep Soundly With The Delicious New Science of SANE Eating/ Jonathan Bailor.—1st ed.
p. cm.
1. Health   2. Weight Loss   3. Cooking   4. Recipes   5. Diet   6. Nutrition
I. Bailor, Jonathan   II. Title.

Manufactured in the United States of America. First Edition.
The information expressed here is intended for educational purposes only. This information is provided with the understanding that neither Jonathan Bailor nor Yopti, LLC nor SANESolution nor affiliates are rendering medical advice of any kind. This information is not intended to supersede or replace medical advice, nor to diagnose, prescribe or treat any disease, condition, illness or injury. It is critical before beginning any eating or exercise program, including those described in this and related works, that readers receive full medical clearance from a licensed physician.

Jonathan Bailor, Yopti, LLC, SANESolution, and affiliates are not liable to anyone or anything impacted negatively, or purported to have been impacted negatively, directly or indirectly, by leveraging this or related information. By continuing to read this and related works the reader accepts all liability and disclaims Jonathan Bailor, Yopti, LLC, SANESolution, and affiliates from any and all legal matters. If these terms are not acceptable, visit SANESolution.com/contact to return this for a full refund.

Christine Lost Over 100 lbs. Now It's <u>Your</u> Turn!

If You Want To Discover The Simple Science Of Slim, Than Grab Your Own SANE Blueprint Today...

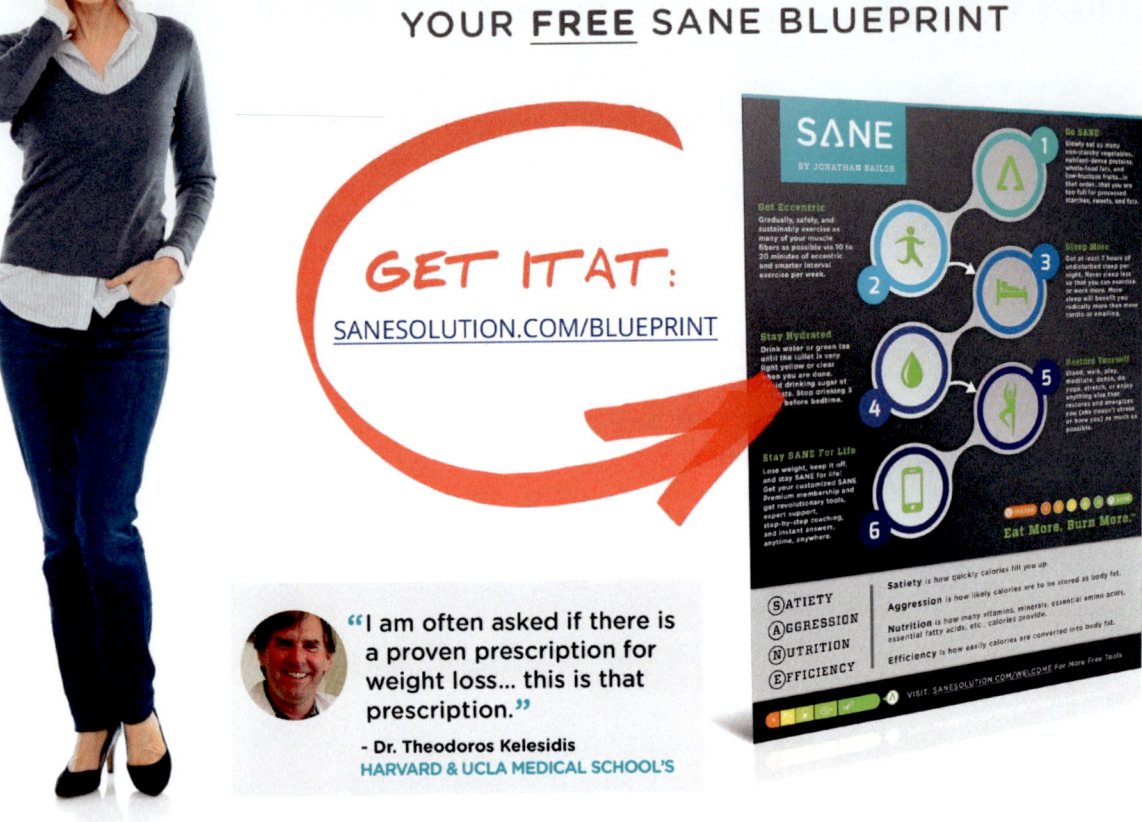

LEARN THE SECRETS TO LOSE 30-100 POUNDS BY EATING MORE & EXERCISING LESS WITH YOUR FREE SANE BLUEPRINT

GET IT AT: SANESOLUTION.COM/BLUEPRINT

"I am often asked if there is a proven prescription for weight loss... this is that prescription."
— Dr. Theodoros Kelesidis
HARVARD & UCLA MEDICAL SCHOOL'S

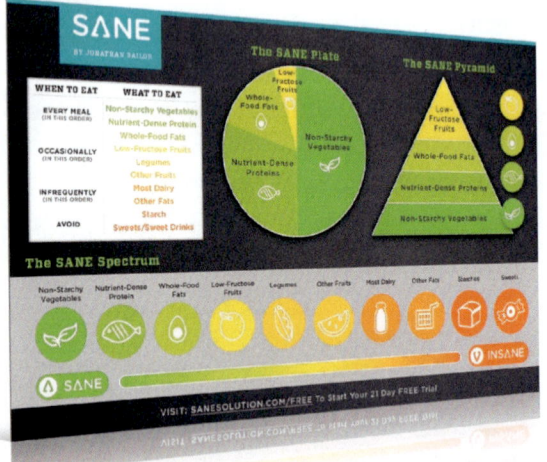
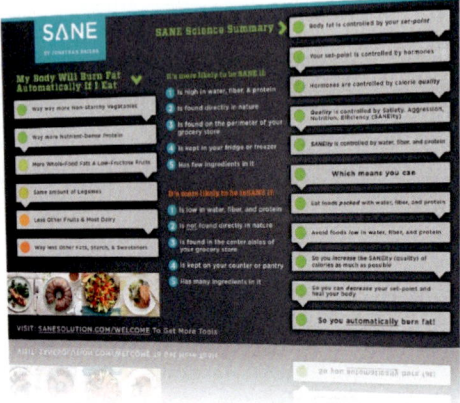

GET YOURS NOW
GO TO: SANESOLUTION.COM/BLUEPRINT

TABLE OF CONTENTS

Introduction 9
Endless Variety and SANE Substitution (vs. Deprivation) 11
SANE Substitution Cheat Sheet 12
MEAT 15
Poultry 16
    Blackened Chicken 16
    Cheesy Chicken 18
    Chicken Tarragon 20
    Chicken Cordon Bleu 22
    Carnival Chicken 24
    Roast Turkey Breast 26
    Cheesy Chicken 28
    Chicken, Bacon & Beef Trifecta 30
    Chicken Citrus 32
    Rosemary Chicken 34
    Rosemary Turkey 36
    Roasted Turkey Breast 38
Beef 40
    Prime Rib 40
    Scrumptious Simple Meatloaf 42
    Barbequed Steak 44
    Herbed Tenderloin 46
    Teriyaki Steak 48
    London Broil 50
    Soy Garlic Flank Steak 52
    Pot Roast 54
    Herbed Tri-Tip 56
    Three Pepper Steak 58
    Marinated Sirloin 60
    Spanish Beef 62

Mushroom Garlic Beef 64
Sirloin Tip Roast 66
Herb Garlic Beef Tenderloin 68
Tri Tip Roast 70

Pork 72
Feta Pork 72
Rosemary Pork Roast 74
Herbed Pork Chops 76
Grilled Pork Chops 78
Pork Burgundy 80
Italian Pork Chops 82
Mustard Soy Tenderloin 84
White Wine Pork Chops 86
Stuffed Pork Chops 88
South American Roast Pork 90
Chili Chops 92

SEAFOOD 94

Cod 96
Lemon Pepper Cod 96
Spinach and Tomatoes Cod 98
Bacon Wrapped Cod 100
Sesame Cod 102

Salmon 104
Salmon Cardamom 104
Hoisin Salmon 106
Cilantro Salmon 108
Moroccan Salmon 110
Scrumptious Baked Salmon 112
Salmon Bake 114
Orange-Ginger Salmon 116
Pan Seared Salmon 118
Garlic Salmon 120

SANE

Free Tools: SANESolution.com/Tools   Superfoods: store.SANESolution.com

- Garlic and Dill Salmon 122
- Spiced Garlic Salmon 124
- Roast Balsamic Salmon 126
- Cedar Salmon 128
- Balsamic Salmon 130
- Garlic Balsamic Salmon 132
- 17 Minute Succulent Salmon 134
- India Salmon 136

Shrimp 138
- Garlic Basil Grilled Shrimp 138
- Italian Shrimp 140
- Herbed Shrimp Scampi 142
- Spiced Shrimp 144
- Shrimp Basil 146
- Bayou Shrimp 148

Tilapia 150
- Old Bay Tilapia 150
- Mustard Tilapia 152
- Tahini Fish 154
- Parmesan Tilapia 156
- Tilapia Feta Florentine 158
- Delicate Parmesan Tilapia 160

Trout 162
- Bacon Trout 162
- Mango Trout 164
- Italian Trout 166
- Mushroom Trout 168
- BBQ Trout 170
- Asian Trout 172

Tuna 174
- 15-Minute Ahi 174
- Horseradish Tuna 176

    Blackened Tuna 178

    Succulent Tuna Steaks 180

    Poached Tuna Steaks 182

    Quick Tuna Steaks 184

    Tuna Citrus 186

    Tuna Tarragon 188

    Wasabi Tuna 190

Other Fish & Seafood 192

    Butter Herb Catfish 192

    Venetian Catfish 194

    Greek Catfish 196

    Crab Encrusted Grouper 198

    Quick Barbecued Sea Bass 200

    Baked Basil Halibut 202

    BBQ Halibut 204

    Ginger Halibut 206

    Pepper and Pesto Mahi Mahi 208

    Cajun Étouffée 210

    Seafood Stew 212

    Grilled Swordfish 214

So Much To Look Forward To... 216

TIP: Not familiar with the SANE Food Group or SANE Serving Sizes?

It's all good! Get everything you need by attending your FREE masterclass at SANESeminar.com and by downloading your FREE tools at SANESolution.com/Tools.

INTRODUCTION

Welcome to the SANE family! Jonathan Bailor here and I want to thank you again for taking time out of your hectic schedule to ensure that **your dinner table is for savoring and smiles, not self-criticism and calorie math**. Eating should be a source of joy and wellness, not shame and sickness. I sincerely hope that our time together will open your eyes to how easy it can be to reach your weight and fitness goals once you break free from the confusing and conflicting outdated theories and lies that have trapped you for so long.

If you only take one thing away from this book let it be this: **Any weight problem you may be experiencing is not your fault!** I know that may sound trite, but it's true. How can you be expected to lose those annoying pounds when all you've been given is outdated science and methods from the 1960's that have been proven NOT to work.

My mission is to not only reshape your body, but it's also to reshape the way you think about weight loss. What that means is I will be here with you every step of the way to provide all the support and tools you need to finally reach your weight loss goals. Whether you need to lose a few extra pounds around your belly, are looking for a **complete body transformation**, want **all-day energy**, or just want to make sense of all the confusing and conflicting health information out there once and for all, you are **finally in the right place!**

> TIP: Be sure to add service@SANESolution.com to your email safe senders list/address book. This ensures you get all your upcoming SANE bonus recipes, tools, and how-to videos.

So if you are ready to stop counting calories... Ready to stop killing yourself with exercise you hate... Ready to end your struggle with weight... and are tired of being hungry and tired...this is your chance. It's time to get off the dieting roller-coaster once and for all. **Are you ready?**

I urge you to make a commitment to yourself to continue this journey. You are worth it. After all, you took action to get this book so that means you are ready and willing to step up and make positive changes. If you follow the simple and scientifically backed principles we teach, **I promise you will lose weight...and keep it off for good.**

You are part of the family now, and I am so excited to have you here as we bust the myths that have been holding you back... perhaps for years. Remember this...**now is your time**, and these are your proven tools for lasting weight loss success. Welcome home.

Can't wait to meet you at SANESolution.com,

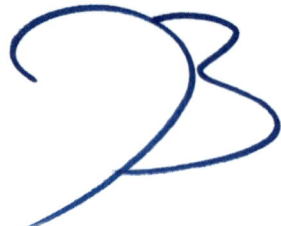

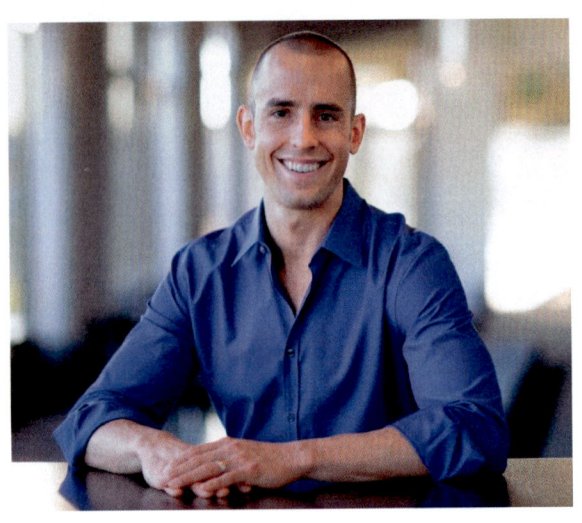

Jonathan Bailor
New York Times Bestselling Author,
SANE Founder, and soon...your
personal weight-loss coach

P.S. Over the years I have found that our most successful members, the ones who have lost 60, 70, even 100 pounds...and kept it off...are the ones who started their personal weight-loss plan on our FREE half-day Masterclass. It's your best opportunity to fall in love with the SANE lifestyle, learn exactly how to start making the simple changes that lead to dramatic body transformations, and get introduced to your new SANE family. **Be sure to reserve your spot now at http://SANESeminar.com.**

Endless Variety and SANE Substitution (vs. Deprivation)

Going SANE isn't about deprivation. It's about enjoying so much good food that you are too full for the sickening stuff. Even better, there are A LOT of delicious recipes that do not require unnatural, fattening, toxic, and addictive ingredients :) In fact, chocolate is the most craved food in the world, and the ingredient that puts the "c" in chocolate—cocoa—is spectacularly SANE.

Keeping "substitution rather than deprivation" principle in mind, you can cook and eat almost anything by making some simple swaps. While these swaps will taste slightly different, they will also make you look and feel completely different—a tradeoff that you will very much enjoy long term. The following cheat sheet will get you started SANEly swapping your way to slimness.

The best thing about this SANE swap approach is that it means that you have access to an endless supply of SANE recipes. All you need to do is find a recipe you like, and then SANEitize it! For example, some of the *SANECertified*™ recipes here were inspired by amazing semi-SANE recipes found around the web. Be sure to check out an ever-growing list of our favorite sites for SANEitizable recipe inspiration at http://bit.ly/InspireSANESubstitution.

> *Inspiration + SANE Substitutions = Endless Variety = :)*

If you would like help with making SANE substitutions, please attend our free interactive masterclass webinar at http://SANESeminar.com.

SANE Substitution Cheat Sheet

inSANE	SANE
Pasta & Rice	- Spaghetti squash/Squoodles - Zucchini noodles/Zoodles - Shirataki noodles - Shredded cabbage - Shaved brussels sprouts - Bean sprouts - Pea shoots - Cauliflower rice - Broccoli and carrot slaw (premade in grocery produce section)
Potatoes	- Mashed cauliflower - Turnips - Eggplant - Squash - Zucchini
Bread, Cookies, Cakes, Pies, Waffles, Pancakes, and Tortillas	- Baked goods made using golden flaxseed meal, coconut flour, almond meal, almond flour, and other nut flours - Low-carb and diabetic breads, tortillas, etc. that contain as few ingredients as possible - Clean Whey Protein - SANE Bars & Energy Bites
Hot and cold cereal	- SANE cereals made with coconut flour, chia, ground flax, and nuts.
Pretzels & chips	- SANE Bake-N-Crisps - Nuts - Seeds - Baked kale chips
Candy Bars, Energy Bars & Drinks, Chocolate	- SANE Bars & Energy Bites

TIP: Not familiar with the SANE Food Group or SANE Serving Sizes?

It's all good! Get everything you need by attending your FREE masterclass at SANESeminar.com and by downloading your FREE tools at SANESolution.com/Tools.

FREE HALF-DAY INTERACTIVE MASTERCLASS WITH NEW YORK TIMES BEST SELLING AUTHOR AND NATURAL WEIGHT-LOSS EXPERT JONATHAN BAILOR

If You Are Ready To Get Off The Yo-Yo Diet Roller-coaster, Then It's Time To Start Your PERSONALIZED WEIGHT LOSS PLAN With Me!

Live Half-Day Seminar Tickets Cost ~~$297~~, But For A Limited Time, You Can Attend Online For FREE!

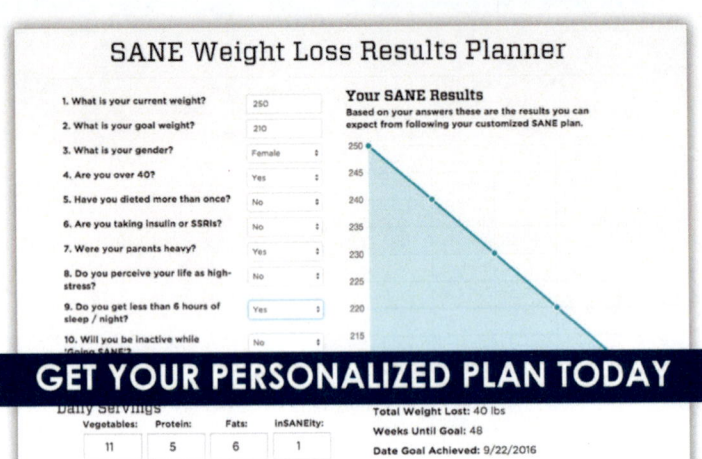

During Our Time Together You Will...

Free yourself from all the confusion and conflicting weight loss information! See the latest science showing you how to get off the yo-yo diet roller-coaster for good, while you overcome emotional eating and cravings.

Learn simple ways to jump-start your motivation today! I'll show you how to effortlessly stick with your new Personalized Weight Loss Plan for lasting results that turn heads and get attention.

Start creating your own personalized weight loss plan--with my help--that will show you exactly how many pounds you can lose per week and even give you an exact date when you will reach your goal weight...without ever counting calories, being hungry, or spending endless hours in the gym!

Discover the one "adjustment" you can make today to increase your energy and ignite your natural fat-burning metabolism so you jump out of bed every morning with confidence.

Crush cravings and end emotional eating with just a few small changes to the types of sweets and fats you are eating. Don't give up what you love, eat more...smarter! Bust the top myths and mistakes that hold you back from losing weight and keeping it off. (You will be relieved when we finally put these lies to rest).

Plus, just for attending you will receive the entire $297 Eat More Lose More Quick Start kit, with videos, cheat sheets, and food guide, for free so you can put this life-changing information to use immediately.

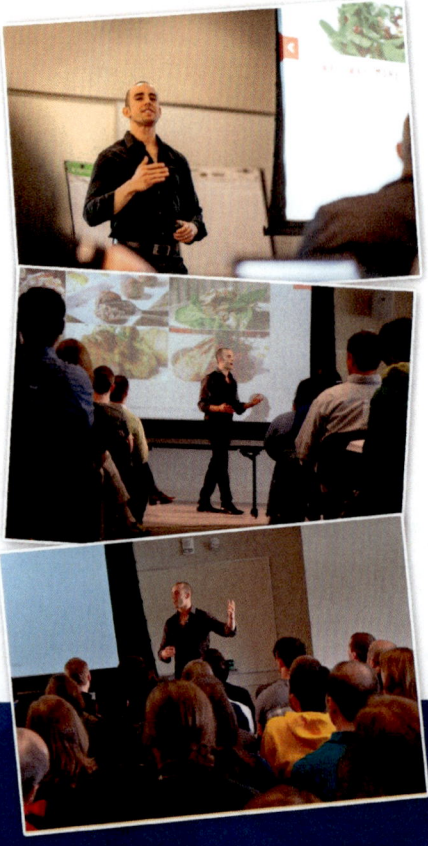

Getting Started Is Easy and Free:
There are many convenient times available

1. Type in this web address: SANESeminar.com
2. Click the button and select a convenient time
3. Enter your information to reserve your seat!

MEAT

Free Tools: SANESolution.com/Tools   Superfoods: store.SANESolution.com

Poultry

Blackened Chicken

Total Time: 20 min
Prep: 10 min
Cook: 10 min

8 Servings
1 Nutrient-Dense Protein Per Serving
1 Whole-Food Fat Per Serving

Ingredients

- 2 teaspoons paprika
- 1/2 teaspoon salt
- 1 teaspoon cayenne pepper
- 1 teaspoon ground cumin
- 1 teaspoon dried thyme
- 1/2 teaspoon ground white pepper
- 1/2 teaspoon onion powder
- 8 skinless, boneless chicken breast halves

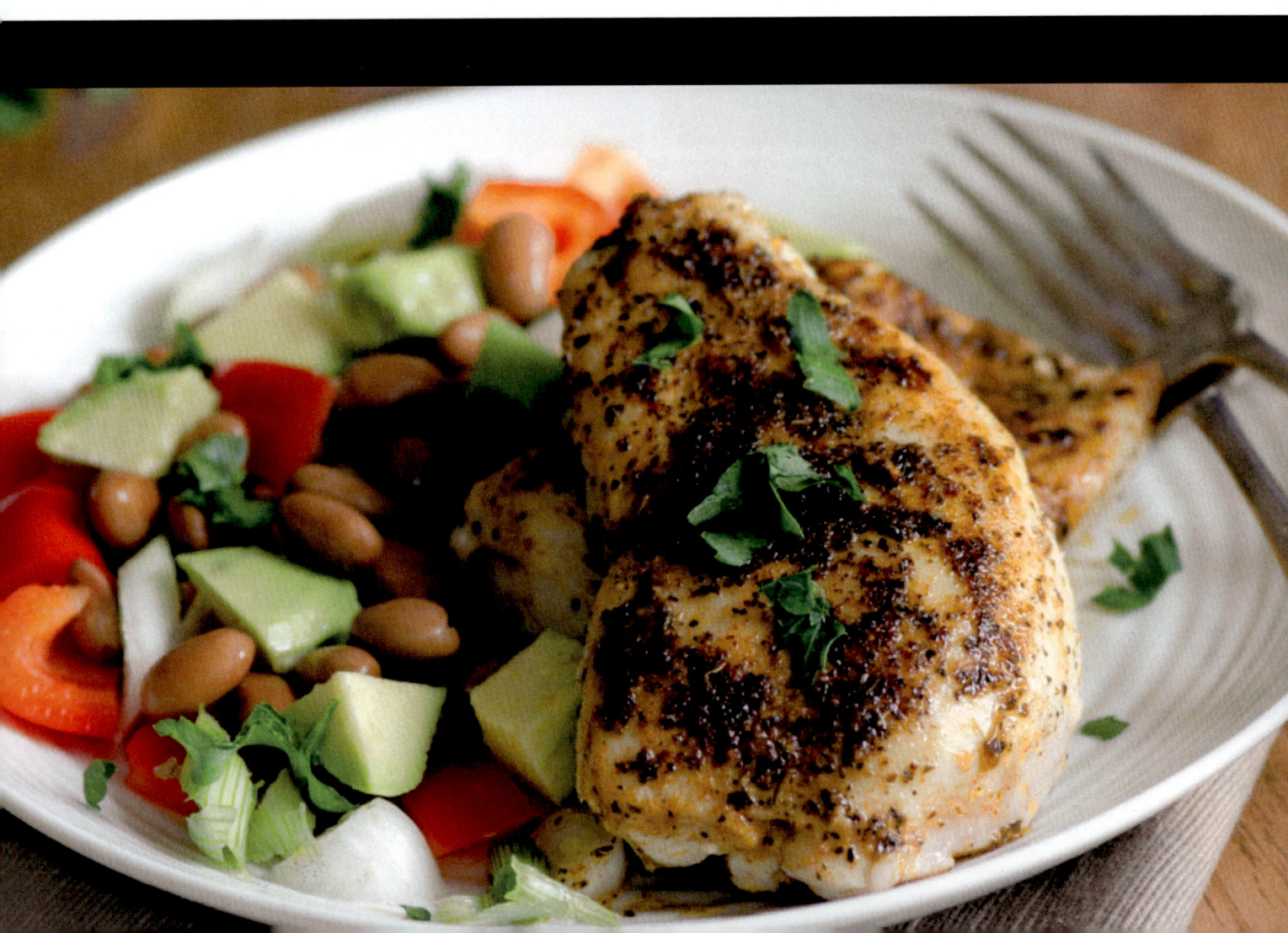

Directions

1. Preheat oven to 350 degrees F (175 degrees C). Lightly grease a baking sheet. Heat a cast iron skillet over high heat for 5 minutes until it is smoking hot.

2. Mix together the paprika, salt, cayenne, cumin, thyme, white pepper, and onion powder. Oil the chicken breasts with cooking spray on both sides, then coat the chicken breasts evenly with the spice mixture.

3. Place the chicken in the hot pan, and cook for 1 minute. Turn, and cook 1 minute on other side. Place the breasts on the prepared baking sheet.

4. Bake in the preheated oven until no longer pink in the center and the juices run clear, about 5 minutes.

SANE   Free Tools: SANESolution.com/Tools   Superfoods: store.SANESolution.com

Cheesy Chicken

Total Time: 45 min
Prep: 15 min
Cook: 30 min

8 Servings
2 Nutrient-Dense Protein Per Serving
1 Whole-Food Fat Per Serving

Ingredients

- 8 skinless, boneless chicken breast halves
- 1/2 pound tomato basil feta cheese, crumbled
- 1/3 cup Italian-style dry bread crumbs, divided

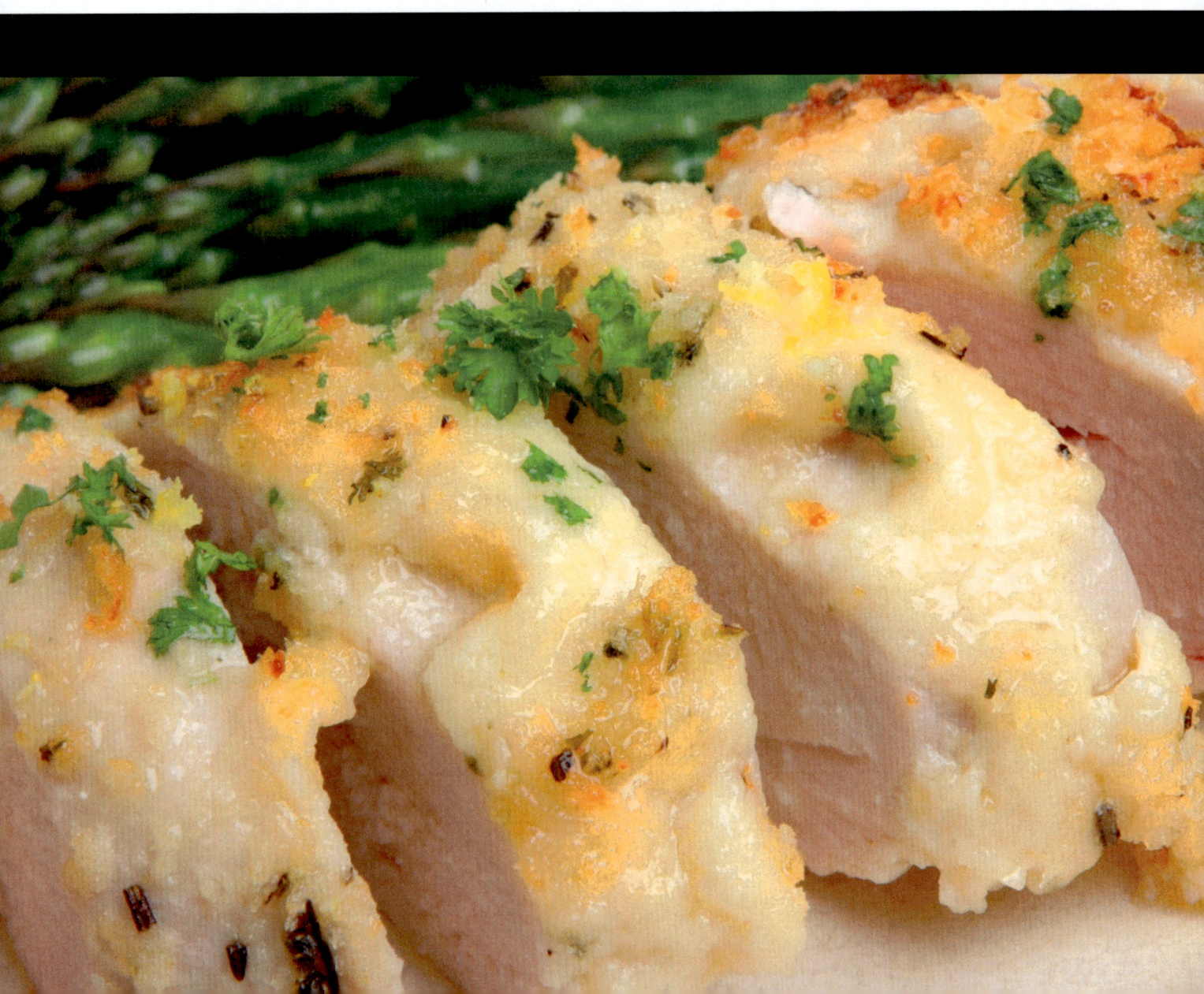

Directions

1. Preheat oven to 350 degrees F (175 degrees C). Lightly grease a 9×13 inch baking dish.

2. Place chicken breasts between 2 pieces of waxed paper. Gently pound chicken with flat side of meat mallet or rolling pin until about 1/4 inch thick; remove wax paper. Place 1 ounce of feta cheese in the center of each chicken breast, and fold in half.

3. Spread 2 tablespoons bread crumbs in the bottom of the prepared baking dish. Arrange chicken in the dish, and top with remaining bread crumbs.

4. Bake 25 to 30 minutes in the preheated oven, or until chicken is no longer pink and juices run clear.

SANE Free Tools: SANESolution.com/Tools   Superfoods: store.SANESolution.com

Chicken Tarragon

Total Time: 45 min
Prep: 15 min
Cook: 30 min

8 Servings
1 Nutrient-Dense Protein Per Serving
2 Whole-Food Fat Per Serving

Ingredients

- 2 tablespoons butter
- 2 tablespoons extra virgin coconut oil
- 8 skinless, boneless chicken breast halves
- salt and pepper to taste
- 1 cup heavy cream
- 2 tablespoons Dijon mustard
- 1 tablespoon and 1 teaspoon chopped fresh tarragon

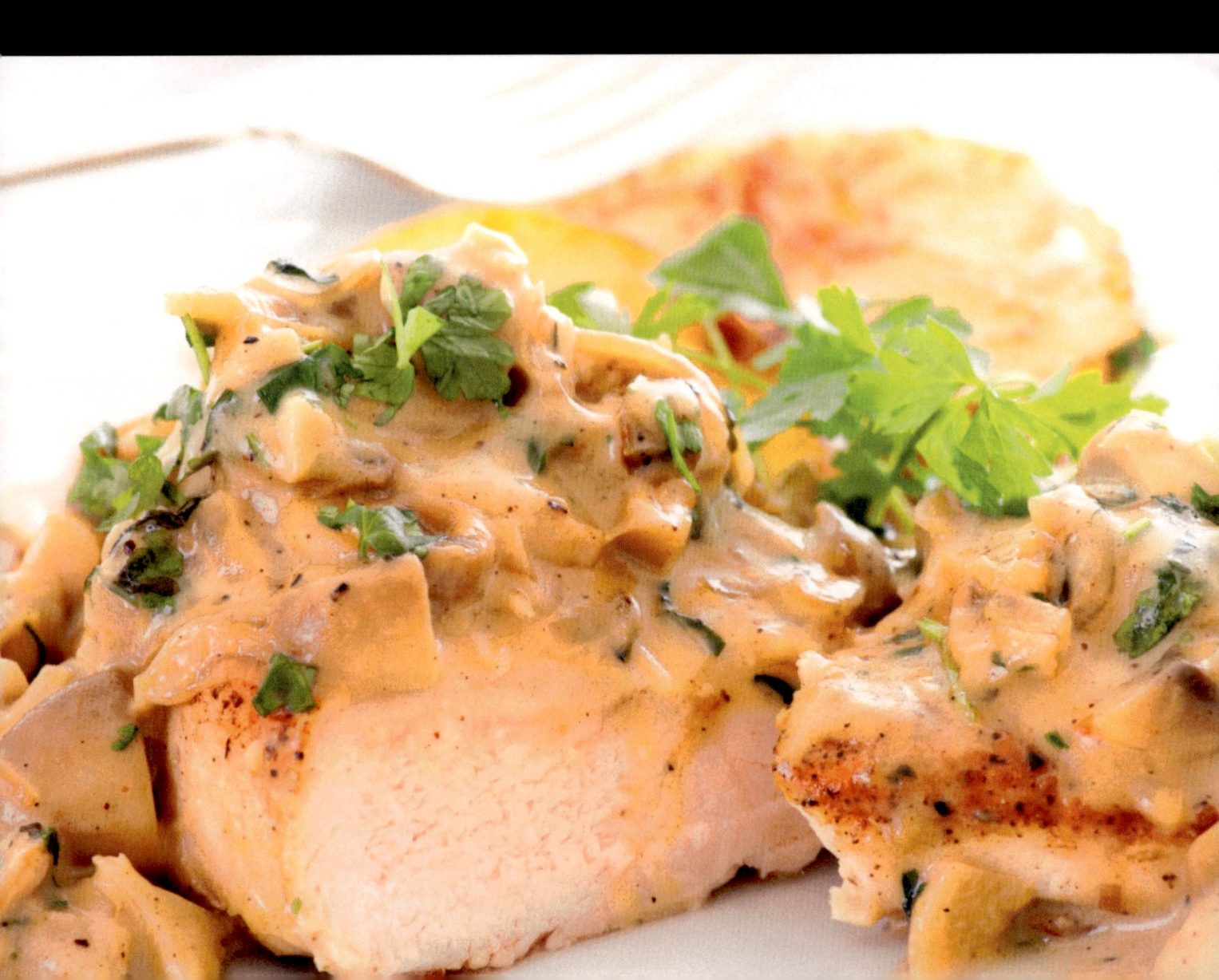

Directions

1. Melt the butter and heat the oil in a skillet over medium-high heat. Season chicken with salt and pepper, and place in the skillet. Brown on both sides. Reduce heat to medium, cover, and continue cooking 15 minutes, or until chicken juices run clear. Set aside and keep warm.

2. Stir cream into the pan, scraping up brown bits. Mix in mustard and tarragon. Cook and stir 5 minutes, or until thickened. Return chicken to skillet to coat with sauce. Drizzle chicken with remaining sauce to serve.

Chicken Cordon Bleu

Total Time: 45 min
Prep: 10 min
Cook: 35 min

8 Servings
2 Nutrient-Dense Protein Per Serving
1 Whole-Food Fat Per Serving
1 Most Dairy Per Serving

Ingredients

- 8 skinless, boneless chicken breast halves
- 1/2 teaspoon salt
- 1/4 teaspoon ground black pepper
- 12 slices Jarlsberg cheese
- 8 slices cooked ham
- 1/2 cup almond meal

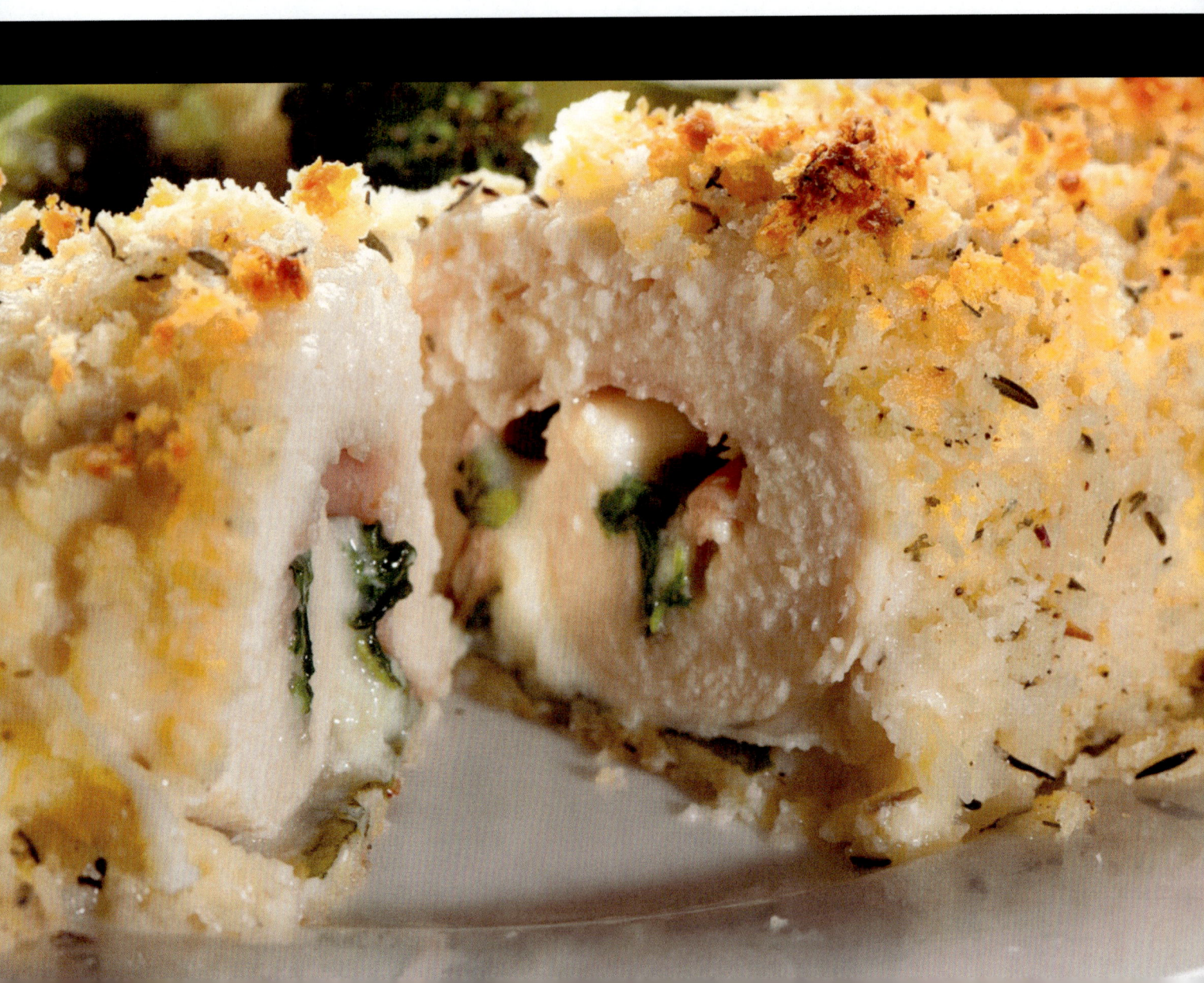

Directions

1. Preheat oven to 350 degrees F (175 degrees C). Coat a 7×11-inch baking dish with nonstick cooking spray.

2. Pound chicken breasts to 1/4-inch thickness. Sprinkle each piece of chicken on both sides with salt and pepper. Place one cheese slice and one ham slice on top of each breast. Roll up each breast and secure with a toothpick. lace in baking dish and sprinkle chicken evenly with almond meal.

3. Bake in preheated oven until chicken breasts are no longer pink in center and juices run clear, 30 to 35 minutes. An instant-read thermometer inserted into the center should read at least 165 degrees F (74 degrees C). Remove from oven and place 1/2 cheese slice on top of each breast. Return to oven and bake until cheese is melted, 3 to 5 minutes. Remove toothpicks and serve immediately.

SANE Free Tools: SANESolution.com/Tools   Superfoods: store.SANESolution.com

Carnival Chicken

Total Time: 25 min
Prep: 5 min
Cook: 20 min

8 Servings
1 Nutrient-Dense Protein Per Serving
1 Whole-Food Fat Per Serving

Ingredients

- 1-1/2 teaspoons salt
- 1/2 teaspoon black pepper
- 1/2 teaspoon cayenne pepper
- 1/4 teaspoon paprika
- 1/2 teaspoon garlic powder
- 1/4 teaspoon onion powder
- 1/2 teaspoon dried thyme
- 1/2 teaspoon dried parsley
- 8 boneless, skinless chicken breast halves
- 1/4 cup butter
- 2 tablespoons extra virgin coconut oil
- 1 tablespoon and 1 teaspoon garlic powder
- 1/4 cup and 2 tablespoons lime juice

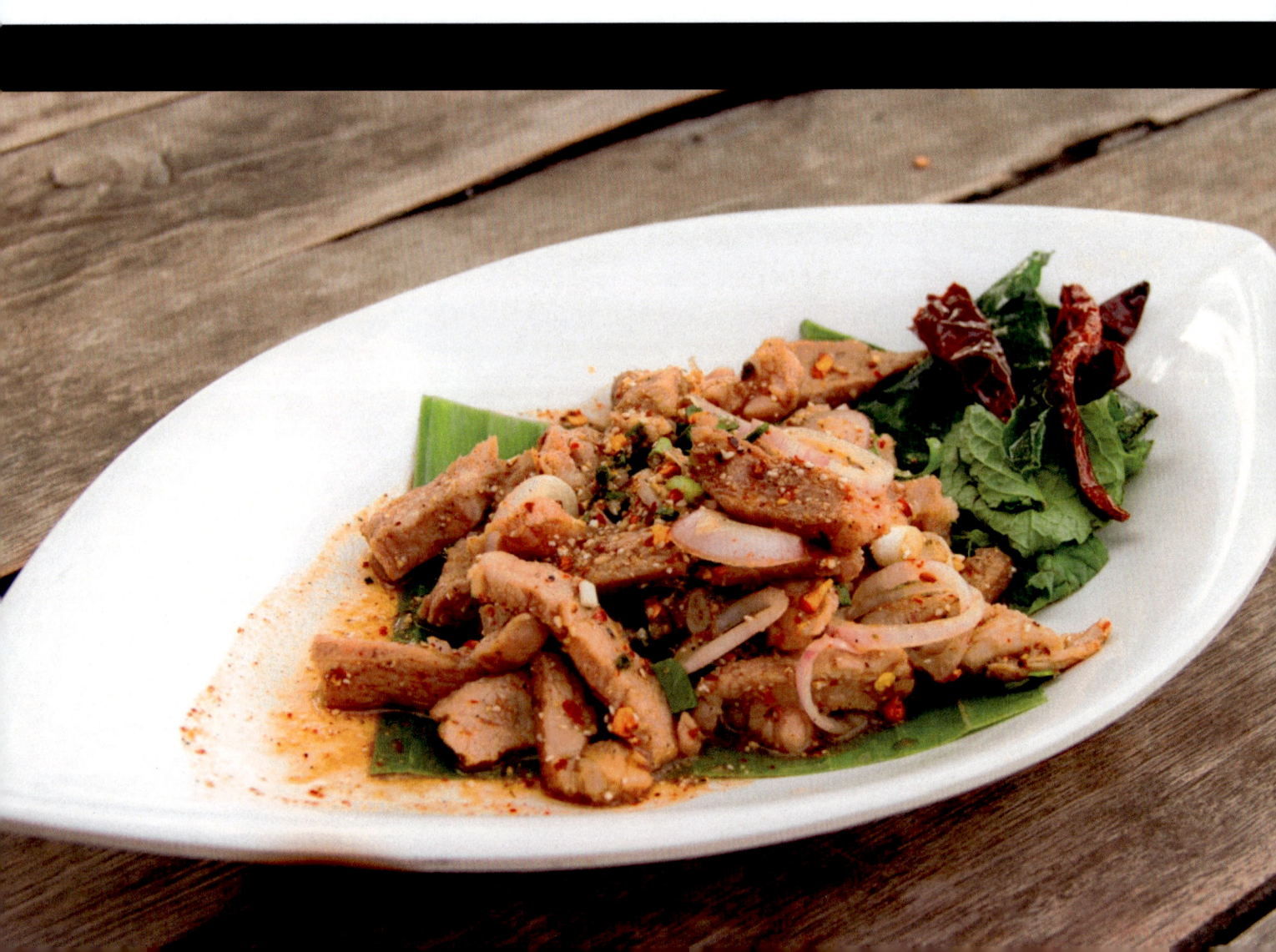

Directions

1. In a small bowl, mix together salt, black pepper, cayenne, paprika, 1/4 teaspoon garlic powder, onion powder, thyme and parsley. Sprinkle spice mixture generously on both sides of chicken breasts.

2. Heat butter and extra virgin coconut oil in a large heavy skillet over medium heat. Saute chicken until golden brown, about 6 minutes on each side. Sprinkle with 2 teaspoons garlic powder and lime juice. Cook 5 minutes, stirring frequently to coat evenly with sauce.

Roast Turkey Breast

Total Time: 1hr 50 min
Prep: 15 min
Cook: 1hr 35 min

8 Servings
2 Nutrient-Dense Protein Per Serving
2 Whole-Food Fat Per Serving

Ingredients

- 1/3 cup butter, softened
- 1-1/4 cloves garlic, minced
- 1-1/4 teaspoons paprika
- 1-1/4 teaspoons Italian seasoning
- 3/4 teaspoon salt-free garlic and herb seasoning blend (such as Mrs. Dash®)
- salt and ground black pepper to taste
- 1-1/4 (3 pound) turkey breast with skin
- 1-1/4 teaspoons minced shallot
- 1 tablespoon and 1 teaspoon butter
- 1-1/4 splashes dry white wine
- 1-1/3 cups chicken stock
- 1/4 cup almond flour
- 2 tablespoons and 2 teaspoons half-and-half (optional)

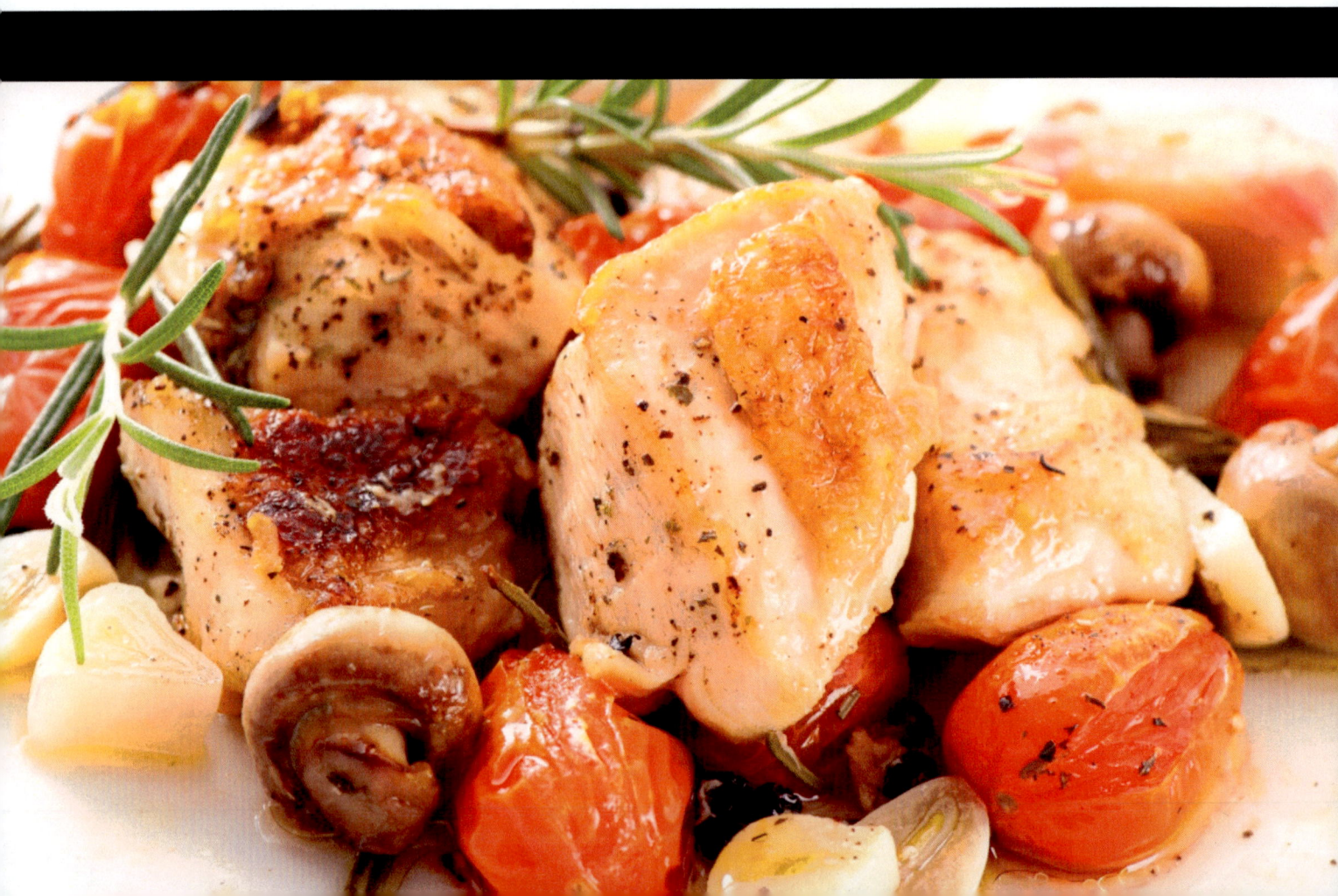

Directions

1. Preheat oven to 350 degrees F (175 degrees C).

2. Mix 1/4 cup butter, garlic, paprika, Italian seasoning, garlic and herb seasoning, salt, and black pepper in a bowl. Place turkey breast with skin side up into a roasting pan. Loosen skin with your fingers; brush half the butter mixture over the turkey breast and underneath the skin. Reserve remaining butter mixture. Tent turkey breast loosely with aluminum foil.

3. Roast in the preheated oven for 1 hour; baste turkey breast with remaining butter mixture. Return to oven and roast until the juices run clear and an instant-read meat thermometer inserted into the thickest part of the breast, not touching bone, reads 165 degrees F (65 degrees C), about 30 more minutes. Let turkey breast rest 10 to 15 minutes before serving.

4. While turkey is resting, transfer pan drippings to a skillet. Skim off excess grease, leaving about 1 tablespoon in skillet. Place skillet over low heat; cook and stir shallot in turkey grease until opaque, about 5 minutes. Melt 1 tablespoon butter in skillet with shallot and whisk in white wine, scraping any browned bits of food from skillet. Whisk in chicken stock and flour until smooth. Bring to a simmer, whisking constantly, until thickened. For a creamier, lighter gravy, whisk in half-and-half.

SANE   Free Tools: SANESolution.com/Tools   Superfoods: store.SANESolution.com

Cheesy Chicken

Total Time: 55 min
Prep: 15 min
Cook: 40 min

8 Servings
2 Nutrient-Dense Protein Per Serving
3 Whole-Food Fat Per Serving
1 Most Dairy Per Serving

Ingredients

- 1/2 cup butter
- 4 cloves garlic, minced
- 3/4 cup almond flour
- 1/2 cup freshly grated Parmesan cheese
- 1 1/2 cups shredded Cheddar cheese
- 1/4 teaspoon dried parsley
- 1/4 teaspoon dried oregano
- 1/4 teaspoon ground black pepper
- 1/8 teaspoon salt
- 8 skinless, boneless chicken breast halves – pounded thin

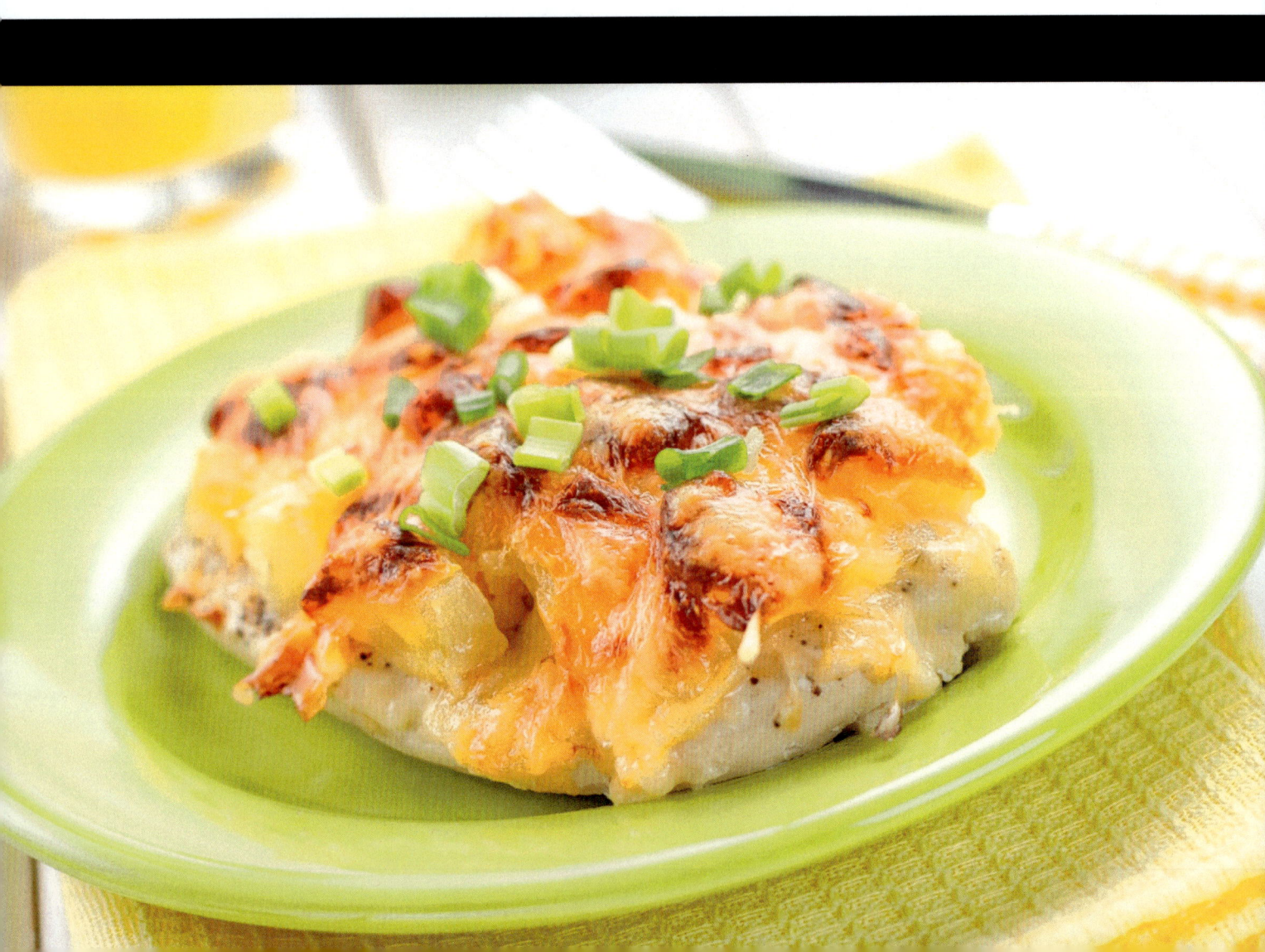

Directions

1. Preheat oven to 350 degrees F (175 degrees C).

2. Melt the butter in a saucepan over low heat, and cook the garlic until tender, about 5 minutes.

3. In a shallow bowl, mix the almond flour, Parmesan cheese, Cheddar cheese, parsley, oregano, pepper, and salt.

4. Dip each chicken breast in the garlic butter to coat, then press into the almond flour mixture. Arrange the coated chicken breasts in a 9×13 inch baking dish. Drizzle with any remaining butter and top with any remaining almond flour mixture.

5. Bake 30 minutes in the preheated oven, or until chicken is no longer pink and juices run clear.

Chicken, Bacon & Beef Trifecta

Total Time: 20 min
Prep: 10 min
Cook: 10 min

8 Servings
2 Nutrient-Dense Protein Per Serving
2 Whole-Food Fat Per Serving
1 Other Fats Per Serving

Ingredients

- 8 slices thin-sliced cooked corned beef
- 8 skinless, boneless chicken breast halves
- 8 slices bacon
- 1-1/4 (10.75 ounce) cans condensed cream of mushroom soup
- 1-1/4 (8 ounce) containers sour cream
- 1-1/4 heads broccoli, broken into florets (optional)

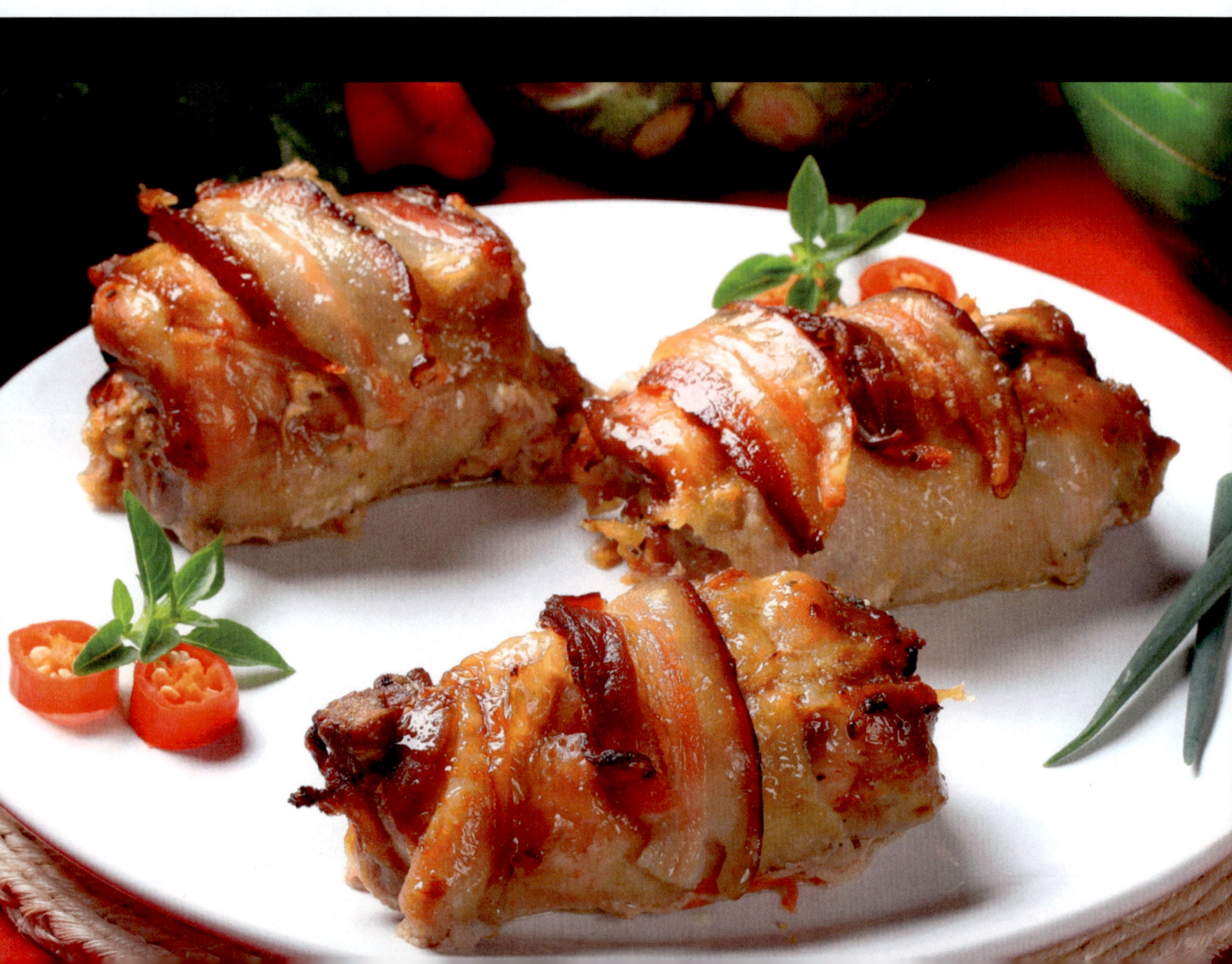

Directions

1. Preheat oven to 325 degrees F (165 degrees C).

2. Wrap 1 corned beef slice around each chicken breast.

3. Wrap a slice of bacon around outside of corned beef wrapping. Secure with toothpicks if needed.

4. Arrange wrapped chicken in a deep baking dish.

5. Arrange broccoli florets around wrapped chicken breasts.

6. Stir cream of mushroom soup and sour cream together in a bowl. Pour the mixture over the chicken and broccoli to completely cover. Cover baking dish with aluminum foil.

7. Bake in preheated oven until chicken is no longer pink in the center and the juices run clear, about 1 1/2 hours. Remove foil from the dish, return to oven, and bake until bacon browns, about 30 more minutes.

SANE Free Tools: SANESolution.com/Tools   Superfoods: store.SANESolution.com

Chicken Citrus

Total Time: 1hr 10 min
Prep: 10 min
Cook: 1hr

8 Servings
2 Nutrient-Dense Protein Per Serving
2 Whole-Food Fat Per Serving

Ingredients

- 1-1/4 (3 pound) whole chicken, rinsed and patted dry
- 1-1/4 grapefruit, cut in half
- 1 tablespoon and 1 teaspoon extra virgin coconut oil
- 3/4 teaspoon seasoned salt

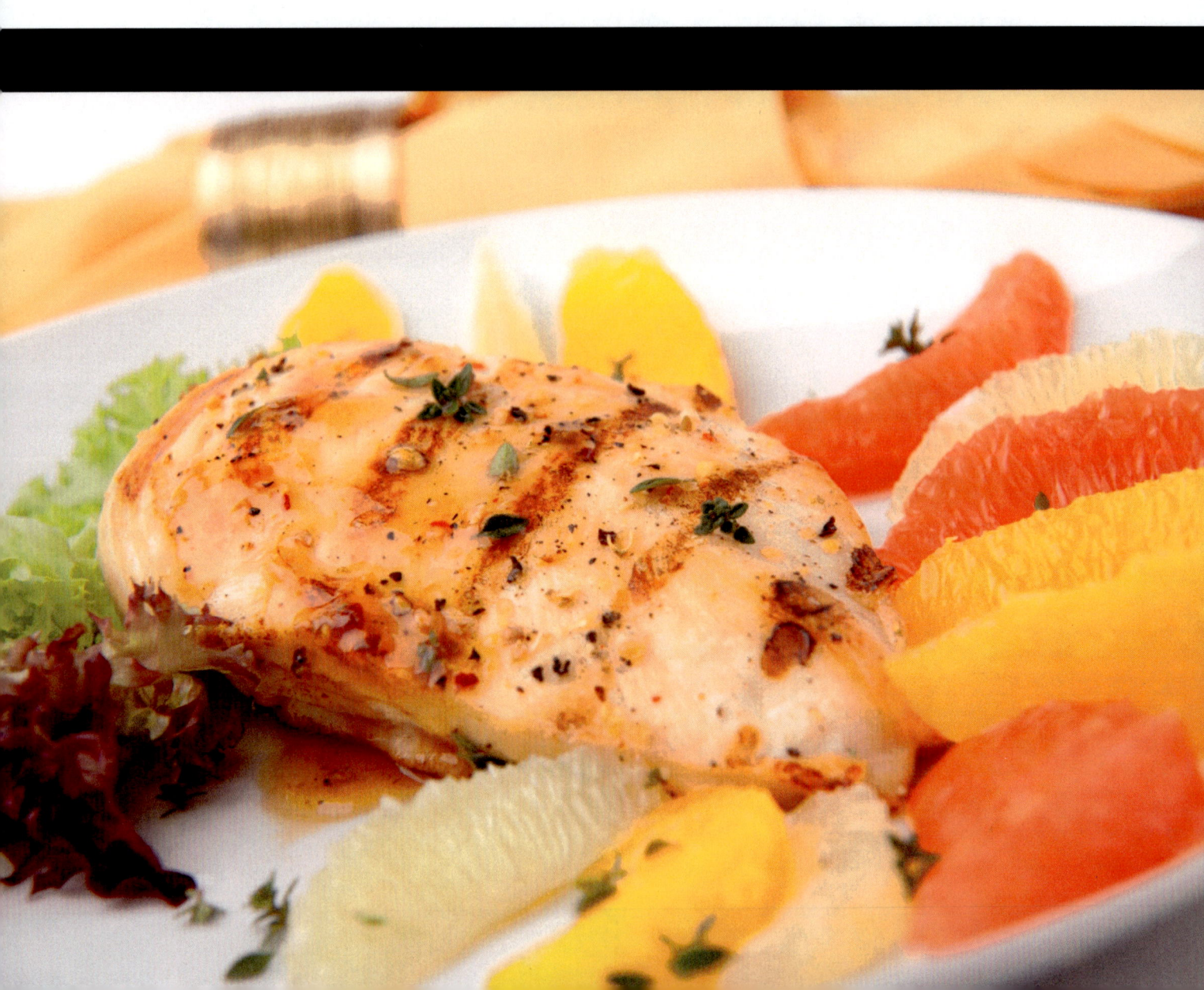

Directions

1. Preheat oven to 400 degrees F (200 degrees C).

2. Place chicken into a roasting pan, and squeeze the juice from the grapefruit halves all over and inside the chicken. Drizzle chicken with extra virgin coconut oil, and sprinkle with seasoned salt. Cover with aluminum foil.

3. Bake in the preheated oven, covered, for 45 minutes; remove foil, and bake until meat is no longer pink at the bone and the juices run clear, about 15 more minutes. An instant-read thermometer inserted into the thickest part of the thigh, near the bone should read 180 degrees F (82 degrees C). Remove the chicken from the oven, cover with a doubled sheet of aluminum foil, and allow to rest in a warm area for 10 minutes before slicing.

SANE   Free Tools: SANESolution.com/Tools   Superfoods: store.SANESolution.com

Rosemary Chicken

Total Time: 2hr 10 min
Prep: 10 min
Cook: 2hr

8 Servings
1 Nutrient-Dense Protein Per Serving
2 Whole-Food Fat Per Serving

Ingredients

- 1-1/4 (3 pound) whole chicken, rinsed
- salt and pepper to taste
- 1-1/4 small onion, quartered
- 1/3 cup chopped fresh rosemary

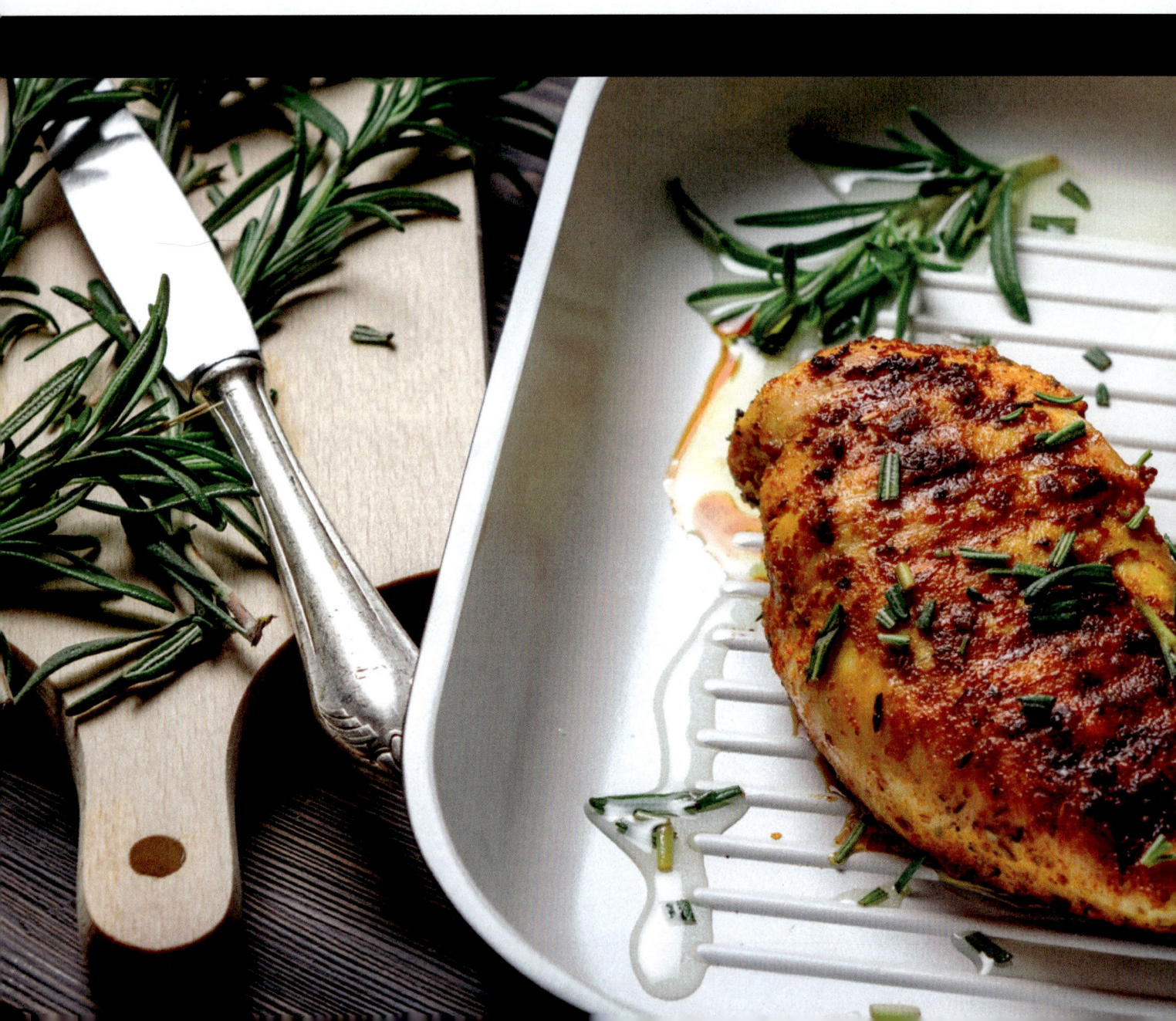

Directions

1. Preheat oven to 350 degrees F (175 degrees C).

2. Season chicken with salt and pepper to taste. Stuff with the onion and rosemary. Place chicken in a 9×13 inch baking dish or roasting dish.

3. Roast in the preheated oven for 2 to 2 1/2 hours, or until chicken is cooked through and juices run clear. Cooking time will vary a bit depending on the size of the bird.

SANE Free Tools: SANESolution.com/Tools   Superfoods: store.SANESolution.com

Rosemary Turkey

Total Time: 4hr 30 min
Prep: 4hr
Cook: 30 min

8 Servings
1 Nutrient-Dense Protein Per Serving
1 Whole-Food Fat Per Serving

Ingredients

- 2 pounds turkey tenderloins
- 1/4 cup and 2 tablespoons soy sauce
- 2 tablespoons Dijon-style prepared mustard
- 1 tablespoon and 1 teaspoon dried rosemary, crushed

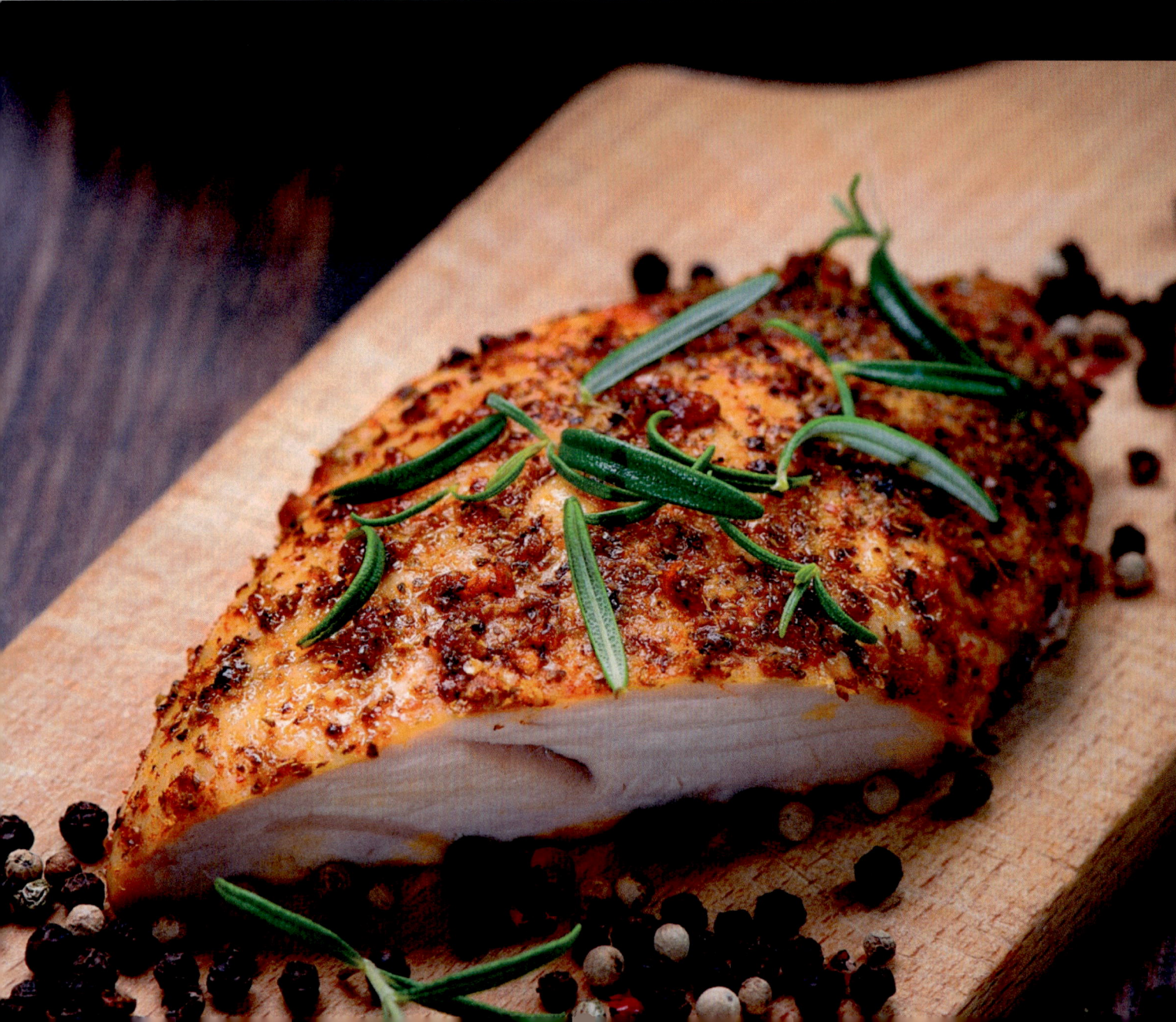

Directions

1. Place the turkey tenderloins in a sealable plastic bag and set aside.

2. In a small bowl combine the soy sauce, mustard and rosemary. Pour over turkey, seal bag and shake to coat. Marinate in the refrigerator for 1 to 4 hours shaking once or twice.

3. Preheat oven on the broiler setting. Remove the turkey from the marinade and place on the rack in the broiler pan. Broil 4 inches from the heat, turning once, for 20 to 22 minutes or until meat is cooked through and when pierced with a fork the juices run clear. Slice and serve with Cranberry Chutney.

SANE   Free Tools: SANESolution.com/Tools   Superfoods: store.SANESolution.com

Roasted Turkey Breast

Total Time: 5hr 10 min
Prep: 10 min
Cook: 5hr

8 Servings
2 Nutrient-Dense Protein Per Serving
2 Whole-Food Fat Per Serving

Ingredients

- 5/8 (8 pound) whole bone-in turkey breast with skin
- 1 cup chicken stock
- 1/4 cup butter, melted
- 1-1/4 teaspoons chicken bouillon granules
- 3/4 teaspoon dried sage
- 3/4 teaspoon dried savory
- 3/4 teaspoon dried rosemary
- 3/4 teaspoon dried thyme

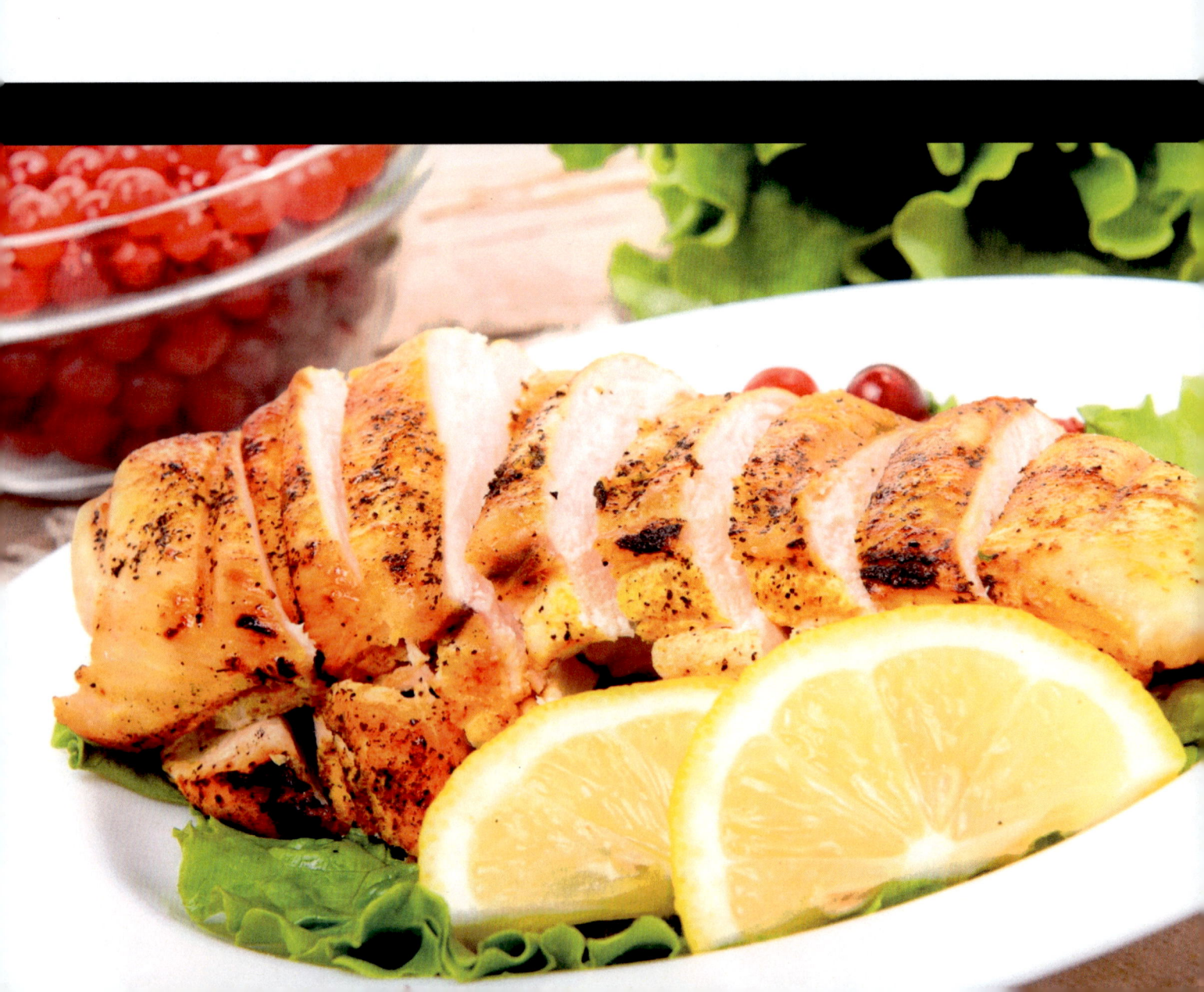

Directions

1. Preheat oven to 350 degrees F (175 degrees C).

2. Loosen the skin from the meat of the turkey breast.

3. Place the turkey breast into a large oven-safe pot or Dutch oven with a lid and pour chicken stock over the meat. Mix melted butter with chicken bouillon granules, sage, savory, rosemary, and thyme in a bowl. Lift the loosened skin and pour slightly more than half the butter-herb mixture under the skin. Pour remaining herb mixture over the skin. Cover the pot.

4. Roast in the preheated oven for 3 hours; flip turkey breast over and roast 1 more hour; flip again and roast until the juices run clear and an instant-read meat thermometer inserted into the thickest part of the breast, not touching bone, reads 180 degrees F (80 degrees C), 1 additional hour (5 hours in all). Baste turkey with pan drippings and let stand 5 to 10 minutes before serving.

SANE Free Tools: SANESolution.com/Tools   Superfoods: store.SANESolution.com

Beef

Prime Rib

Total Time: 4hr 40 min
Prep: 10 min
Cook: 4hr 30 min

8 Servings
3 Nutrient-Dense Protein Per Serving
2 Whole-Food Fat Per Serving

Ingredients

- 2-2/3 cups coarse kosher salt
- 5-1/4 pounds prime rib roast
- 1 tablespoon and 1 teaspoon ground black pepper
- 1 tablespoon and 1 teaspoon seasoning salt

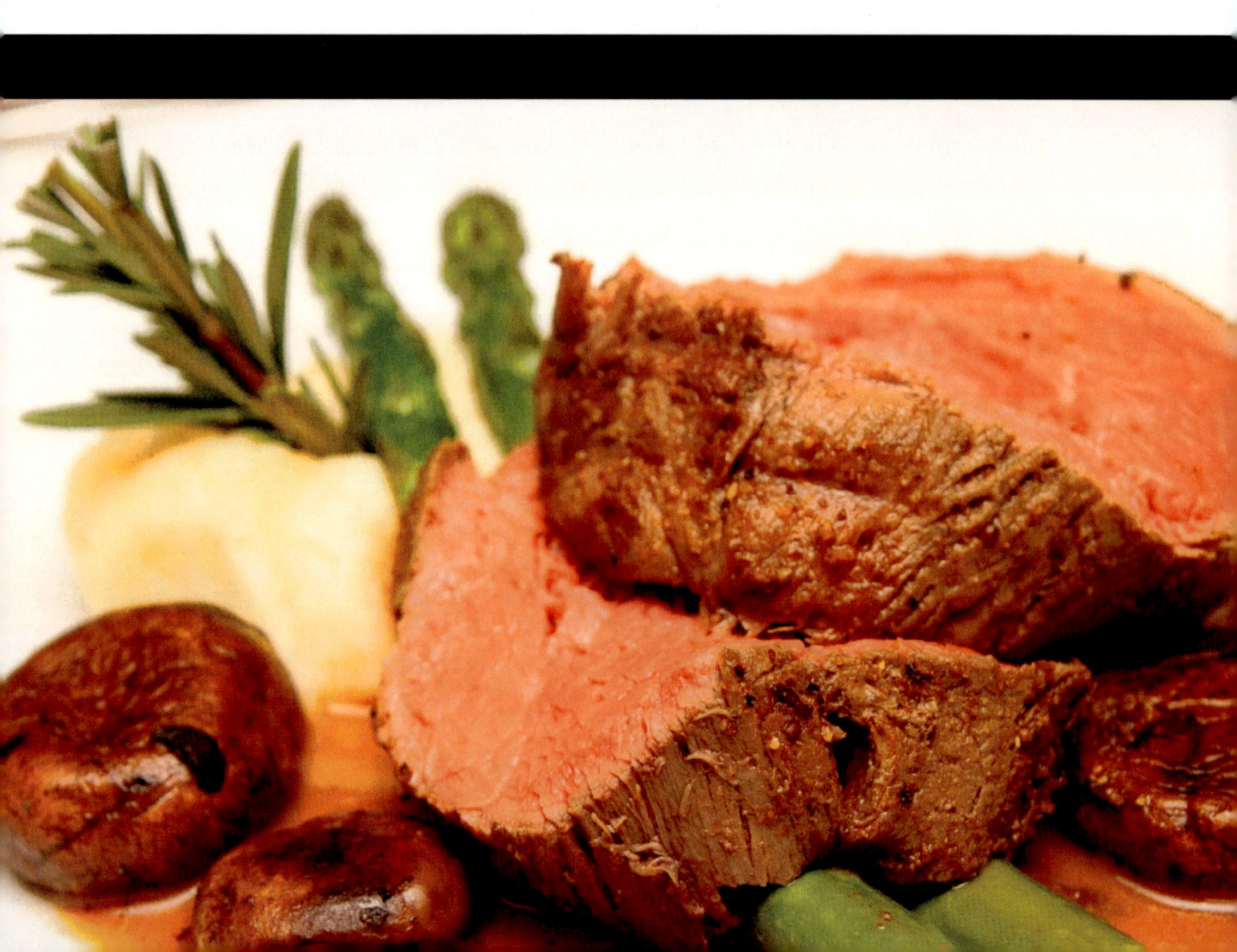

Directions

1. Preheat oven to 210 degrees F (100 degrees C).

2. Cover the bottom of a roasting pan with a layer of kosher salt. Place the roast, bone side down, on the salt. Season the meat with the ground black pepper and seasoning salt, then cover completely with kosher salt.

3. Roast in preheated oven for 4 to 5 hours, or until the internal temperature of the meat reaches 145 degrees F (63 degrees C).

4. Remove from oven and let rest for 30 minutes. This sets the juices and makes the roast easier to carve. (Note: Be sure to remove all the salt from the roast before serving.)

SANE

Free Tools: SANESolution.com/Tools Superfoods: store.SANESolution.com

Scrumptious Simple Meatloaf

Total Time: 55 min
Prep: 10 min
Cook: 45 min

8 Servings
1 Nutrient-Dense Protein Per Serving
2 Whole-Food Fat Per Serving
1 Most Dairy Per Serving

Ingredients

- 2 pounds lean ground beef
- 2/3 cup crushed buttery round crackers
- 1 cup shredded Cheddar cheese
- 1-1/4 (1 ounce) packages dry onion soup mix
- 2-3/4 eggs, beaten
- 1/3 cup ketchup
- 2 tablespoons and 2 teaspoons steak sauce

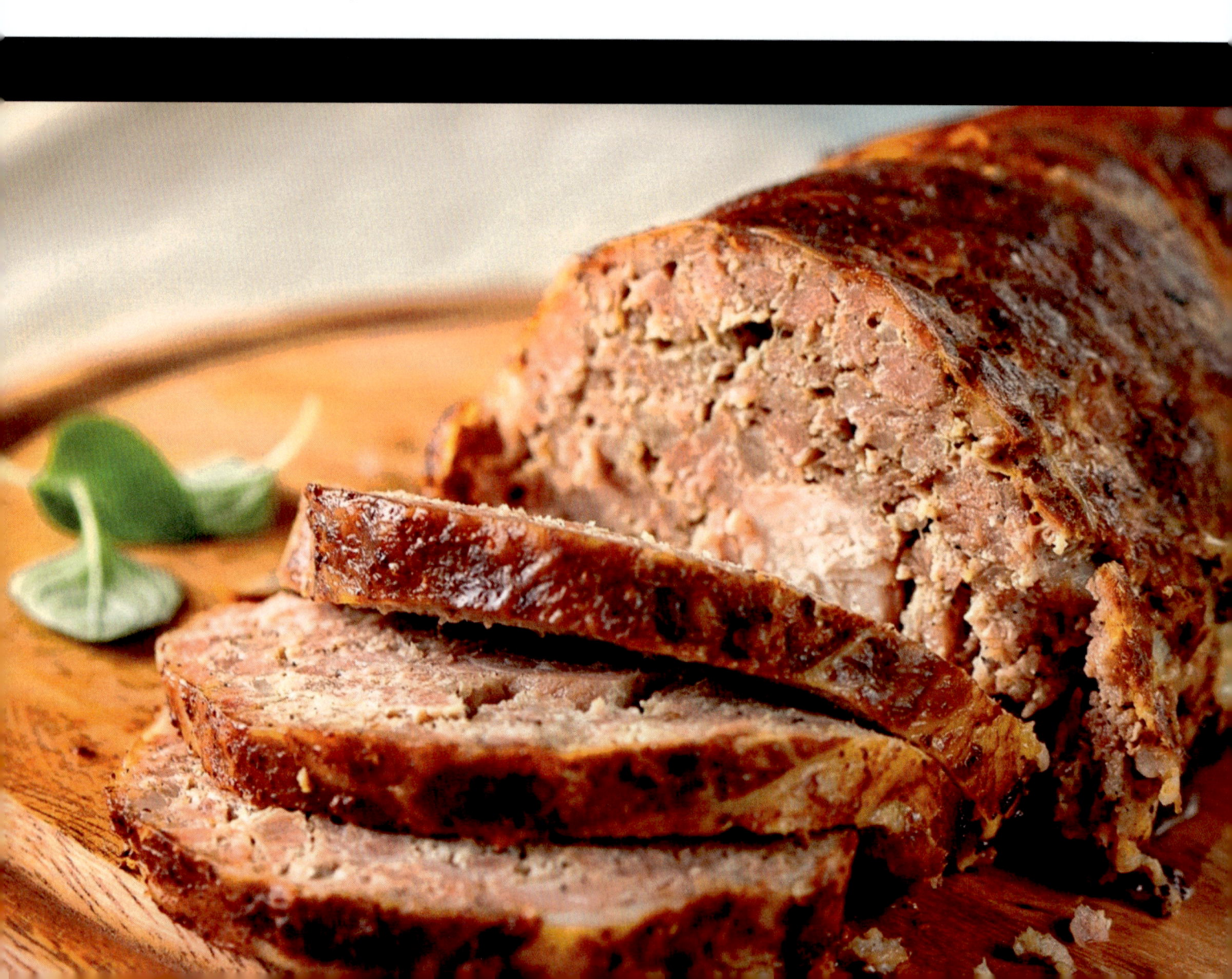

Directions

1. Preheat oven to 350 degrees F (175 degrees C).

2. Stir the ground beef, crushed crackers, Cheddar cheese, and onion soup mix in a large bowl until well combined. Whisk the eggs, ketchup, and steak sauce in a separate bowl until smooth. Mix the eggs into the meat until evenly combined, if the mixture seems too dry, add a little water. Press into a 9×5 inch loaf pan.

3. Bake in preheated oven until the meatloaf reaches 160 degrees F (71 degrees C) and is no longer pink in the center, 45 to 60 minutes.

SANE

Free Tools: SANESolution.com/Tools   Superfoods: store.SANESolution.com

Barbequed Steak

Total Time: 25 min
Prep: 15 min
Cook: 10 min

8 Servings
1 Nutrient-Dense Protein Per Serving
3 Whole-Food Fat Per Serving

Ingredients

- 1/3 cup soy sauce
- 1/4 cup honey
- 2 tablespoons and 2 teaspoons distilled white vinegar
- 3/4 teaspoon ground ginger
- 3/4 teaspoon garlic powder
- 2/3 cup extra virgin coconut oil
- 2 pounds flank steak

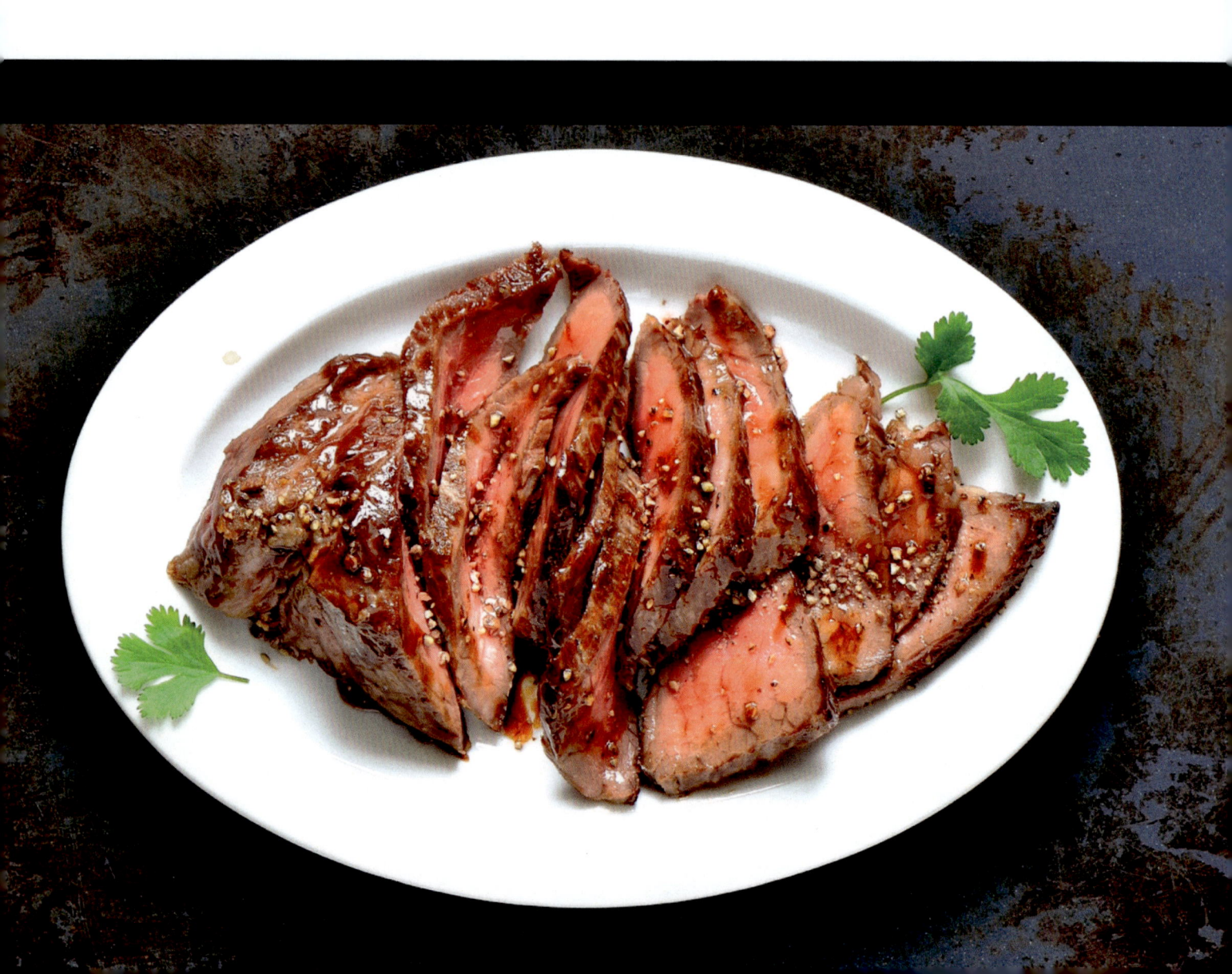

Directions

1. In a blender, combine the soy sauce, honey, vinegar, ginger, garlic powder, and melted extra virgin coconut oil.

2. Lay steak in a shallow glass or ceramic dish. Pierce both sides of the steak with a sharp fork. Pour marinade over steak, then turn and coat the other side. Cover, and refrigerate 8 hours, or overnight.

3. Preheat grill for high heat.

4. Place grate on highest level, and brush lightly with oil. Place steaks on the grill, and discard marinade. Grill steak for 10 minutes, turning once, or to desired doneness.

SANE   Free Tools: SANESolution.com/Tools   Superfoods: store.SANESolution.com

HERBED TENDERLOIN

Total Time: 28 min
Prep: 20 min
Cook: 8 min

8 Servings
2 Nutrient-Dense Protein Per Serving
1 Whole-Food Fat Per Serving

Ingredients

- 4 (8 ounce) fillets beef tenderloin
- 24 fresh sage leaves
- 4 cloves garlic, cut into sixths
- 16 fresh thyme sprigs
- salt and ground black pepper to taste

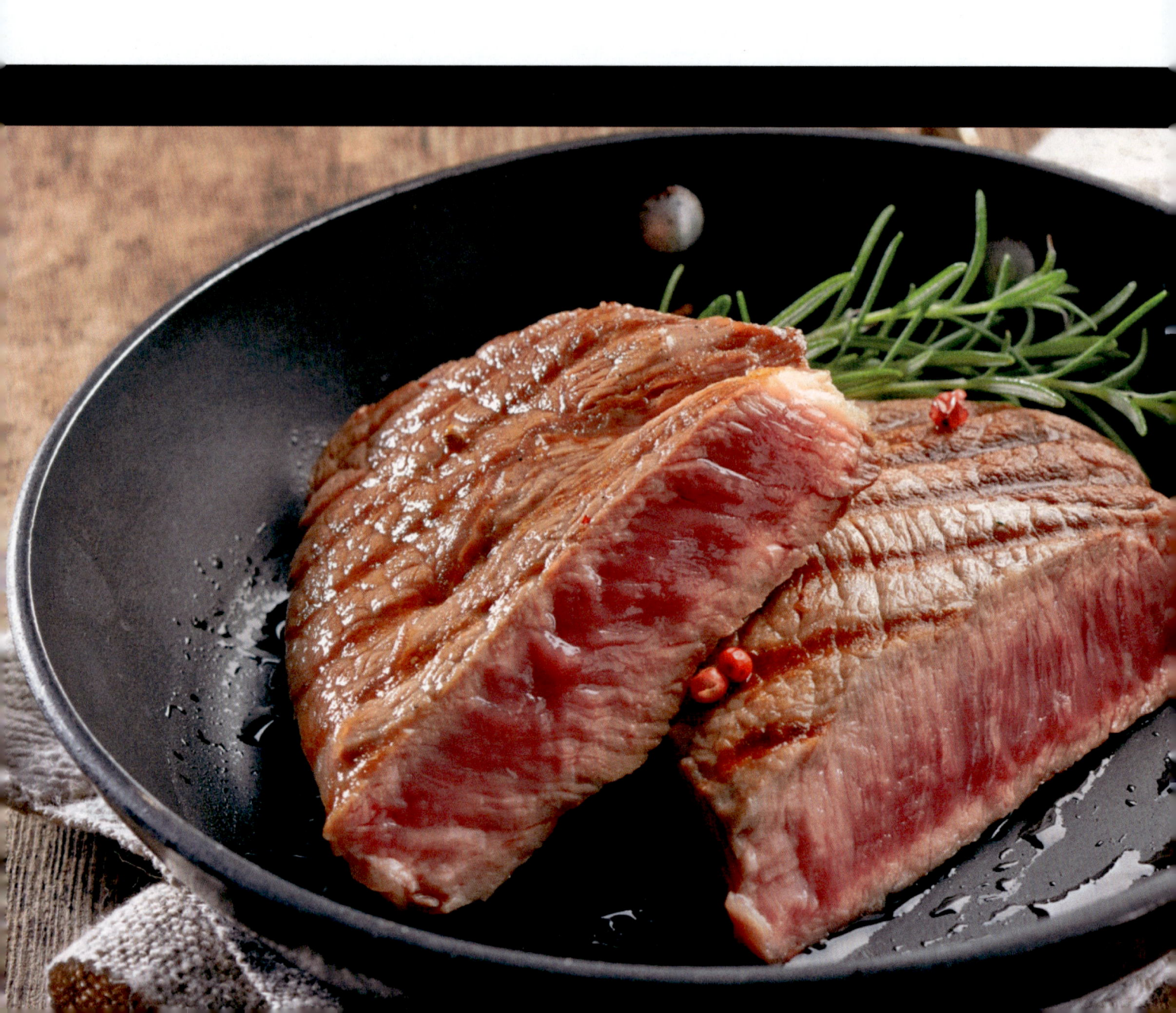

Directions

1. Cut a few 2-inch slits in the side of the fillet; stuff the sage leaves and garlic pieces into the slits. Wrap the thyme sprigs around the fillet. Store in refrigerator to allow the meat to absorb the flavors for 4 to 12 hours.

2. Preheat an outdoor grill for medium heat; lightly oil the grate. Cut the tenderloin in half and season with salt and pepper.

3. Cook the fillets 4 to 6 minutes per side, until no longer pink, or to desired doneness.

Teriyaki Steak

Total Time: 45 min
Prep: 30 min
Cook: 15 min

8 Servings
2 Nutrient-Dense Protein Per Serving
2 Whole-Food Fat Per Serving

Ingredients

- 4 (16 ounce) beef sirloin steaks
- 1/2 cup dark beer
- 1/4 cup teriyaki sauce
- 1/4 cup brown sugar
- 1 teaspoon seasoned salt
- 1 teaspoon black pepper
- 1 teaspoon garlic powder

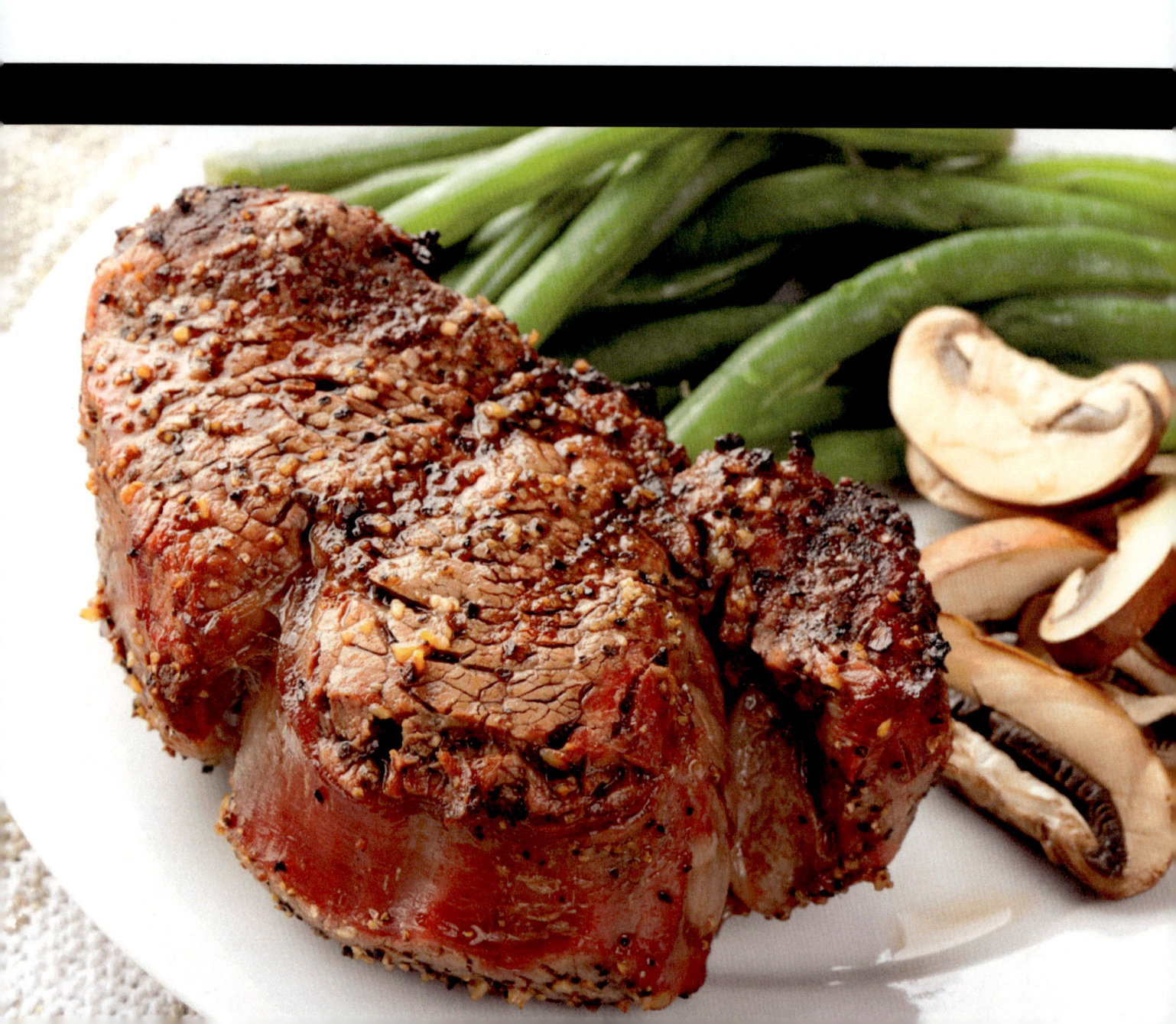

Directions

1. Preheat grill for high heat.

2. Use a fork to poke holes all over the surface of the steaks, and place steaks in a large baking dish. In a bowl, mix together beer, teriyaki sauce, and brown sugar. Pour sauce over steaks, and let sit about 5 minutes. Sprinkle with 1/2 the seasoned salt, pepper, and garlic powder; set aside for 10 minutes. Turn steaks over, sprinkle with remaining seasoned salt, pepper, and garlic powder, and continue marinating for 10 more minutes.

3. Remove steaks from marinade. Pour marinade into a small saucepan, bring to a boil, and cook for several minutes.

4. Lightly oil the grill grate. Grill steaks for 7 minutes per side, or to desired doneness. During the last few minutes of grilling, baste steaks with boiled marinade to enhance the flavor and ensure juiciness.

London Broil

Total Time: 45 min
Prep: 30 min
Cook: 15 min

8 Servings
2 Nutrient-Dense Protein Per Serving
2 Whole-Food Fat Per Serving

Ingredients

- 1 clove garlic, minced
- 1 teaspoon salt
- 3 tablespoons soy sauce
- 1 tablespoon ketchup
- 1 tablespoon extra virgin coconut oil
- 1/2 teaspoon ground black pepper
- 1/2 teaspoon dried oregano
- 4 pounds flank steak

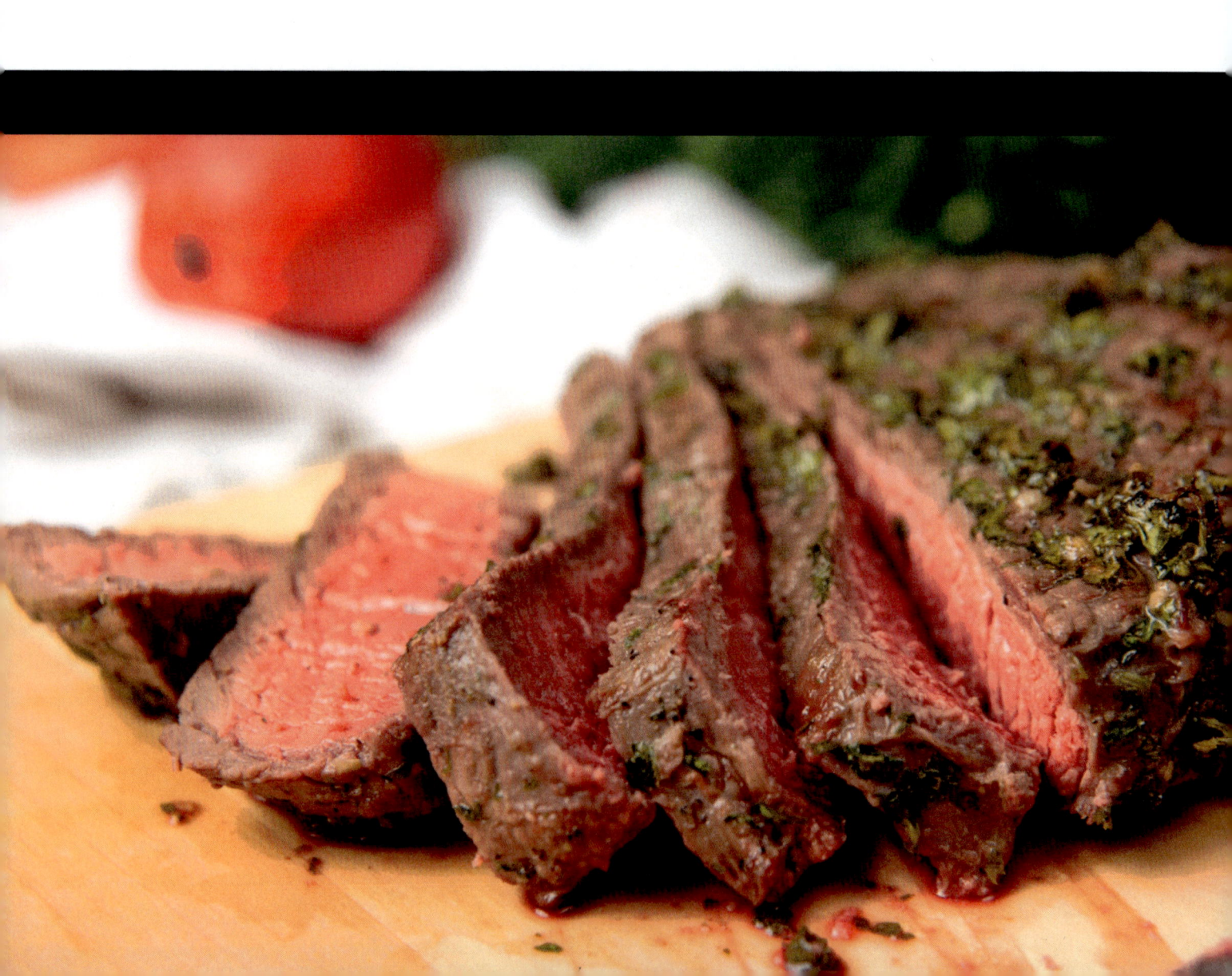

Directions

1. In a small bowl, mix together garlic, salt, soy sauce, ketchup, melted extra virgin coconut oil, black pepper and oregano.

2. Score both sides of the meat, diamond cut, about 1/8 inch deep. Rub garlic mixture into both sides of the meat. Wrap tightly in aluminum foil, and refrigerate for 5 to 6 hours, or overnight. Flip meat every few hours.

3. Preheat an outdoor grill for high heat, and lightly oil grate.

4. Place meat on the prepared grill. Cook for 3 to 7 minutes per side, or to desired doneness.

SANE Free Tools: SANESolution.com/Tools   Superfoods: store.SANESolution.com

Soy Garlic Flank Steak

Total Time: 35 min
Prep: 15 min
Cook: 20 min

8 Servings
1 Nutrient-Dense Protein Per Serving
1 Whole-Food Fat Per Serving

Ingredients

- 2/3 cup soy sauce
- 2 tablespoons and 2 teaspoons brown sugar
- 2 tablespoons and 2 teaspoons lemon juice
- 2 tablespoons and 2 teaspoons extra virgin coconut oil
- 2-3/4 cloves garlic, minced
- 1 tablespoon and 1 teaspoon minced onion
- 1-1/4 teaspoons ground ginger
- 3/4 teaspoon black pepper
- 2 pounds beef flank steak

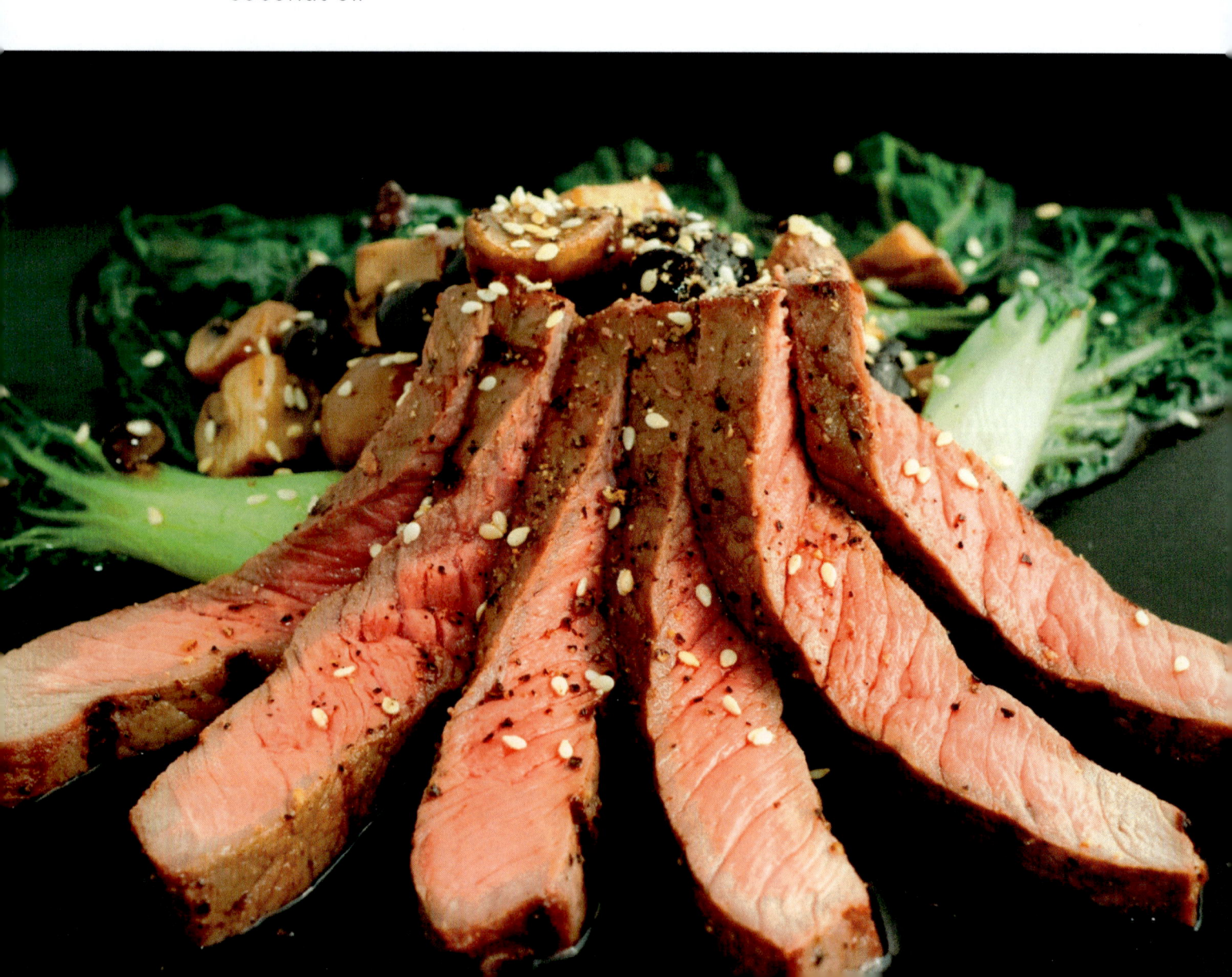

Directions

1. In a shallow bowl, combine soy sauce, brown sugar, lemon juice, melted extra virgin coconut oil, garlic, onion, ginger and pepper. Coat steak with marinade, cover, and refrigerate for at least 6 hours.

2. Preheat an outdoor grill for high heat, and lightly oil grate.

3. Grill steak for 7 to 8 minutes per side, or to desired doneness.

SANE

Free Tools: SANESolution.com/Tools　　Superfoods: store.SANESolution.com

Pot Roast

Total Time: 3hr 15 min
Prep: 15 min
Cook: 3hr

8 Servings
1 Nutrient-Dense Protein Per Serving
2 Whole-Food Fat Per Serving

Ingredients

- 1/3 cup almond meal
- ground black pepper to taste
- 2-1/4 pounds rump roast
- 2 tablespoons and 2 teaspoons butter
- 3/8 (1 ounce) envelope dry onion soup mix
- 5/8 (10.75 ounce) can condensed cream of mushroom soup
- 1/3 cup dry vermouth

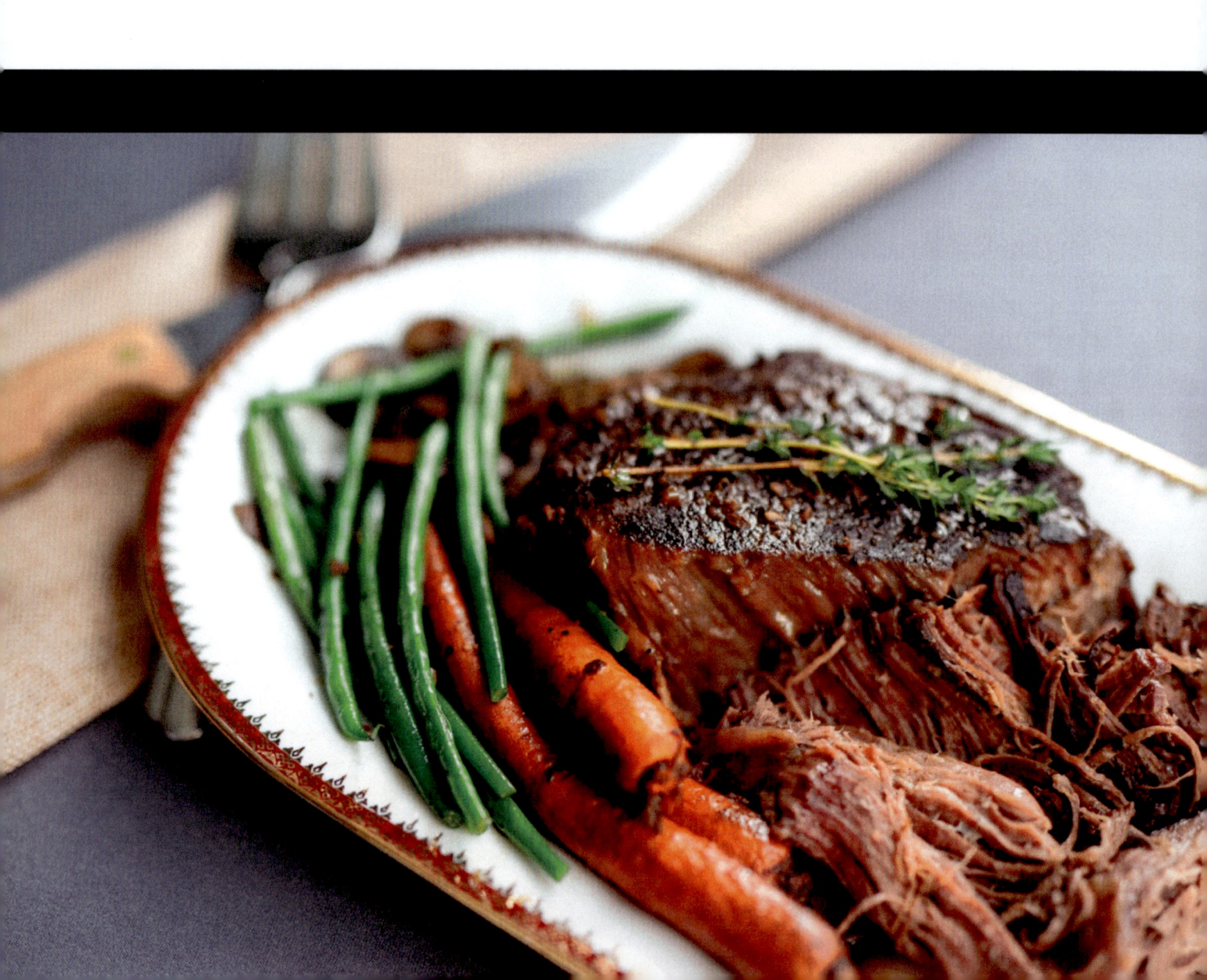

Directions

1. Preheat oven to 325 degrees F (165 degrees C).

2. In a large mixing bowl, combine the almond meal and black pepper to taste. Dredge the rump roast in the flour and cover evenly. Shake off excess.

3. In a large pot over medium/high heat, melt the butter and brown the roast on all sides. Place in a 4 quart casserole dish with lid.

4. In a small bowl, combine the soup mix, mushroom soup, and vermouth or white wine; pour over roast.

5. Cover and bake in preheated oven for 3 hours or until desired doneness.

Herbed Tri-Tip

Total Time: 2hr
Prep: 15 min
Cook: 1hr 45 min

8 Servings
1 Nutrient-Dense Protein Per Serving
1 Whole-Food Fat Per Serving

Ingredients

- 2-1/2 teaspoons salt
- 1-1/4 teaspoons garlic salt
- 1/2 teaspoon celery salt
- 1/4 teaspoon ground black pepper
- 1/4 teaspoon onion powder
- 1/4 teaspoon paprika
- 1/4 teaspoon dried dill
- 1/4 teaspoon dried sage
- 1/4 teaspoon crushed dried rosemary
- 3/4 (2 1/2 pound) beef tri-tip roast

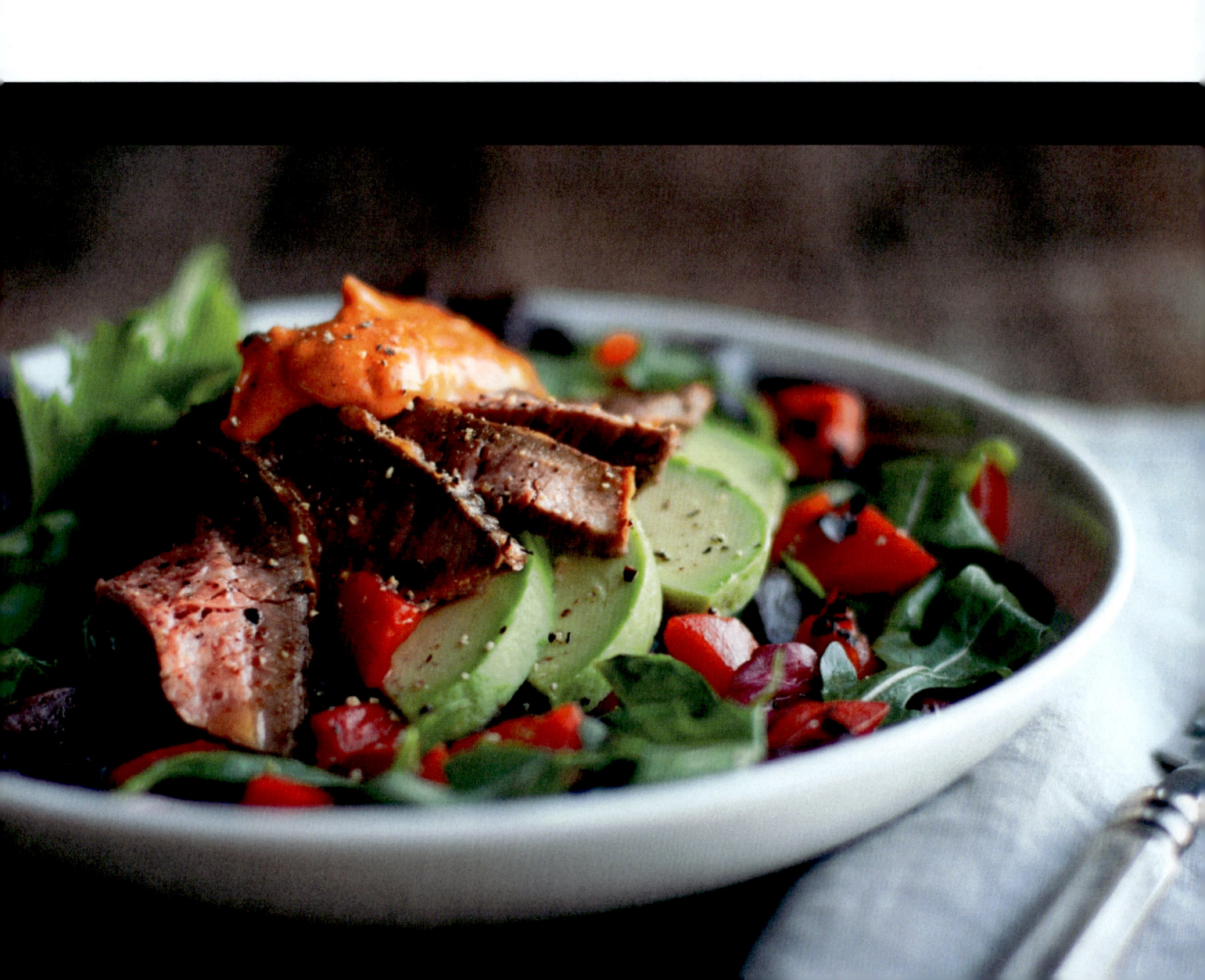

Directions

1. Mix together the salt, garlic salt, celery salt, black pepper, onion powder, paprika, dill, sage, and rosemary in a bowl. Store in an airtight container at room temperature until ready to use.

2. Use a damp towel to lightly moisten the roast with water, then pat with the prepared rub. Refrigerate for a minimum of 2 hours, up to overnight, for the flavors to fully come together.

3. Preheat an outdoor grill for high heat and lightly oil grate.

4. Place the roast onto the preheated grill and quickly cook until brown on all sides to sear the meat, then remove. Reset the grill for medium-low indirect heat (if using charcoal, move coals to the outside edges of the grill pit).

5. Return the roast to the grill, and cook, turning occasionally, until the desired degree of doneness has been reached, about 1 1/2 hours for medium-well. Remove from the grill and cover with aluminum foil. Allow to rest for 10 minutes before carving across the grain in thin slices to serve.

Three Pepper Steak

Total Time: 15 min
Prep: 5 min
Cook: 10 min

8 Servings
1 Nutrient-Dense Protein Per Serving
2 Whole-Food Fat Per Serving

Ingredients

- 1 tablespoon and 1 teaspoon smoked paprika
- 2-3/4 teaspoons salt
- 1-1/4 teaspoons brown sugar
- 2-3/4 teaspoons chili powder
- 1-1/4 teaspoons chipotle chile powder
- 3/4 teaspoon ground black pepper
- 3/4 teaspoon garlic powder
- 3/4 teaspoon onion powder
- 3/4 teaspoon ground cumin
- 2-3/4 pounds flat iron steaks

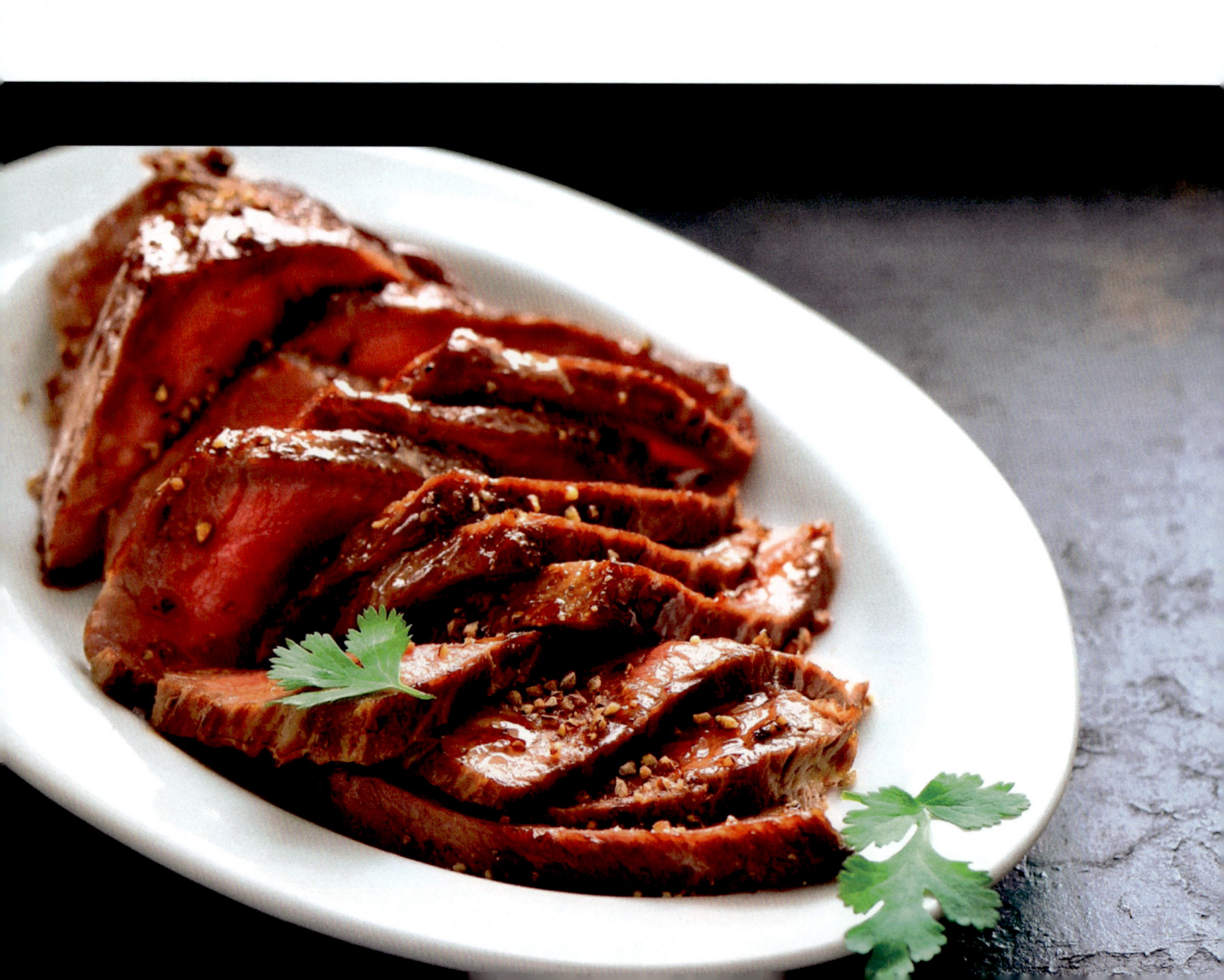

Directions

1. Stir together the paprika, salt, sugar, chili powder, chipotle powder, black pepper, garlic powder, onion powder, and cumin in a small bowl until blended. Rub the seasoning mix all over the flat iron steaks, then wrap them tightly with plastic wrap. Marinate in the refrigerator 2 to 8 hours (the longer the better).

2. Preheat an outdoor grill for medium-high heat, and lightly oil grate.

3. Cook the steaks on the preheated grill until cooked to your desired degree of doneness, about 4 minutes per side for medium. Allow the steaks to rest for 5 minutes in a warm location before slicing.

Marinated Sirloin

Total Time: 15 min
Prep: 5 min
Cook: 10 min

8 Servings
2 Nutrient-Dense Protein Per Serving
2 Whole-Food Fat Per Serving

Ingredients

- 1/4 cup and 2 tablespoons extra virgin coconut oil
- 1/4 cup minced onion
- 2 tablespoons lemon juice
- 2 tablespoons Worcestershire sauce
- 2 tablespoons soy sauce
- 2 teaspoons garlic powder
- 1 teaspoon ground black pepper
- 3 pounds sirloin steak

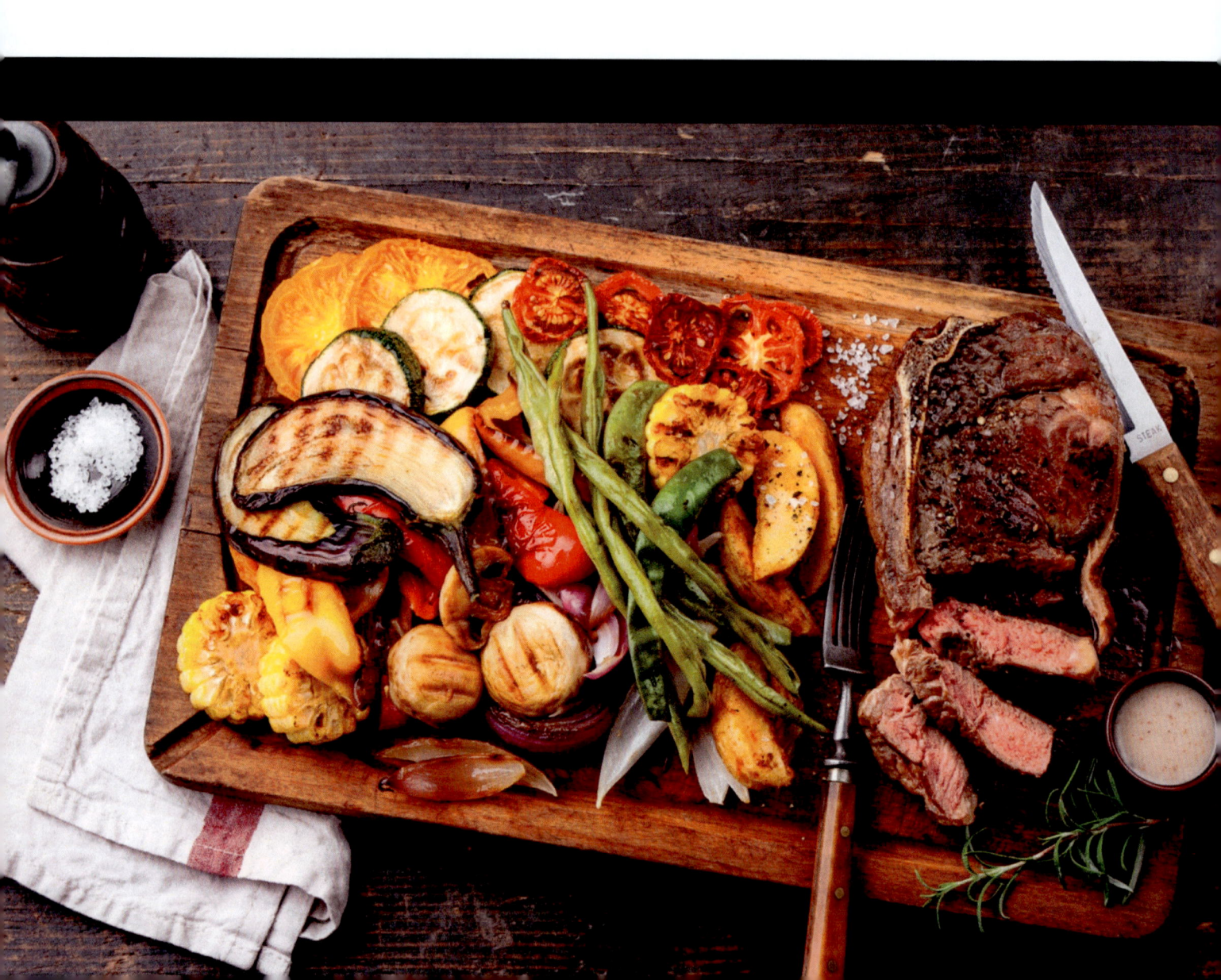

Directions

1. Whisk extra virgin coconut oil, onion, lemon juice, Worcestershire sauce, soy sauce, garlic powder, and pepper in a bowl until marinade is well mixed. Place elk steak in a large resealable plastic bag and pour marinade over meat. Coat meat with marinade, squeeze out excess air, and seal bag. Marinate in the refrigerator for at least 4 hours, turning occasionally.

2. Preheat grill for medium heat and lightly oil the grate. Drain elk steak and discard marinade.

3. Cook steaks on the preheated grill until they are beginning to firm and are hot and slightly pink in the center, 5 minutes per side. An instant-read thermometer inserted into the center should read 140 degrees F (60 degrees C).

SPANISH BEEF

Total Time: 15 min
Prep: 10 min
Cook: 5 min

8 Servings
1 Nutrient-Dense Protein Per Serving
2 Whole-Food Fat Per Serving

Ingredients

- 1/2 cup sherry vinegar
- 1/2 cup extra virgin coconut oil
- 1/4 cup Dijon mustard
- 1/4 tablespoon smoked paprika
- 8 cloves garlic, minced (optional)
- salt and ground black pepper to taste
- 4 pounds very thin flank steak

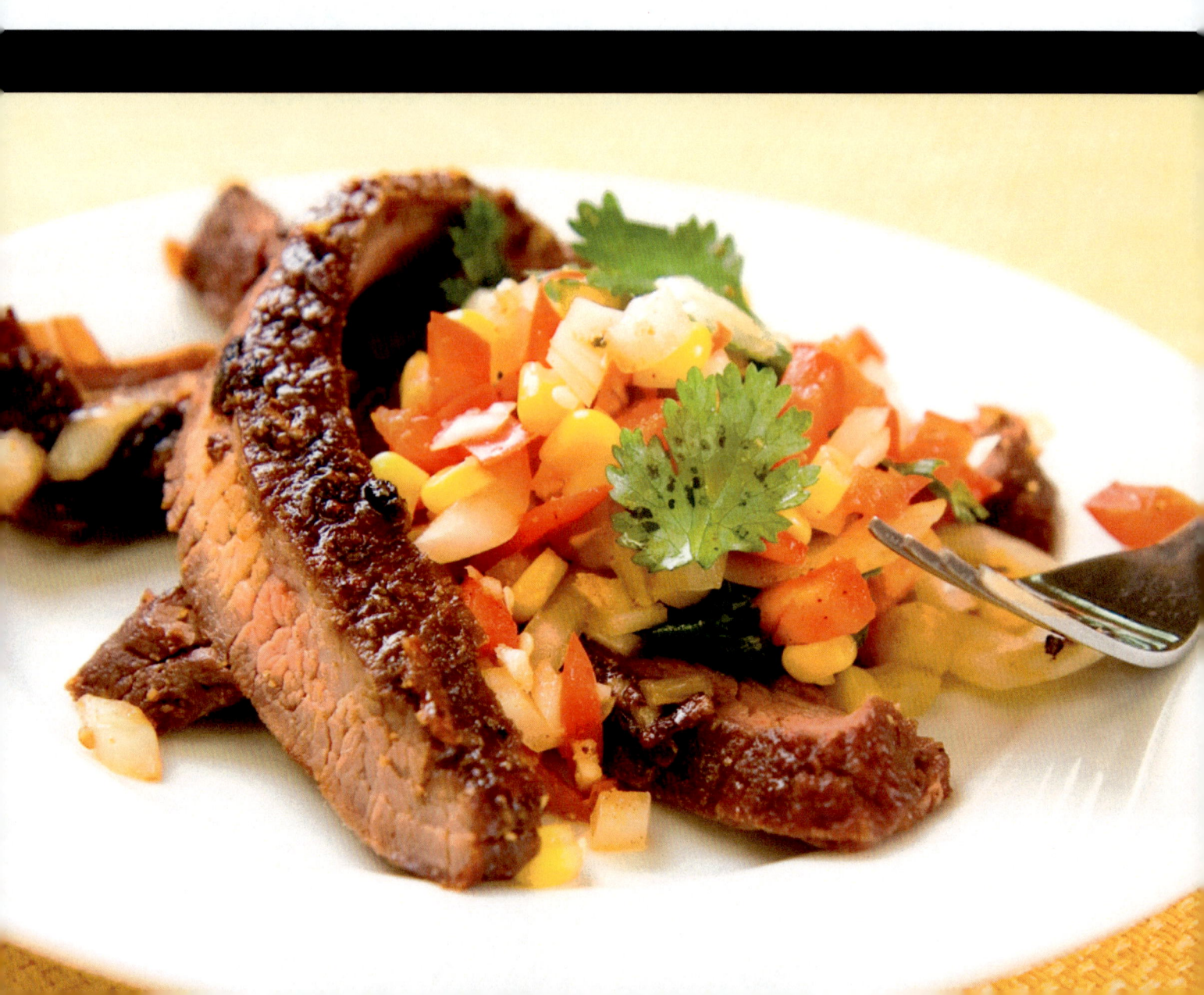

Directions

1. Preheat an outdoor grill for high heat, and lightly oil the grate.

2. Whisk sherry vinegar, extra virgin coconut oil, mustard, paprika, garlic, salt, and pepper together in a large bowl. Place steak in marinade and turn to coat. Marinate at room temperature for 30 minutes.

3. Cook steak on the preheated grill, turning once, until each side is browned, steak is beginning to firm, and is hot and slightly pink in the center, about 2 minutes per side. An instant-read thermometer inserted into the center should read 140 degrees F (60 degrees C). Transfer steak to a plate and let rest for 5 to 10 minutes before slicing.

Mushroom Garlic Beef

Total Time: 20 min
Prep: 10 min
Cook: 10 min

8 Servings
2 Nutrient-Dense Protein Per Serving
2 Whole-Food Fat Per Serving

Ingredients

- 1/4 cup and 2 tablespoons butter
- 8 (7 ounce) beef tenderloin steaks (1 1/2 inches thick)
- 4 cups sliced baby portabella mushrooms
- 8 cloves garlic, finely chopped
- 1/4 cup dry white wine or beef broth
- 2 (9 ounce) pouches Progresso™ Recipe Starters™ creamy portabella mushroom cooking sauce

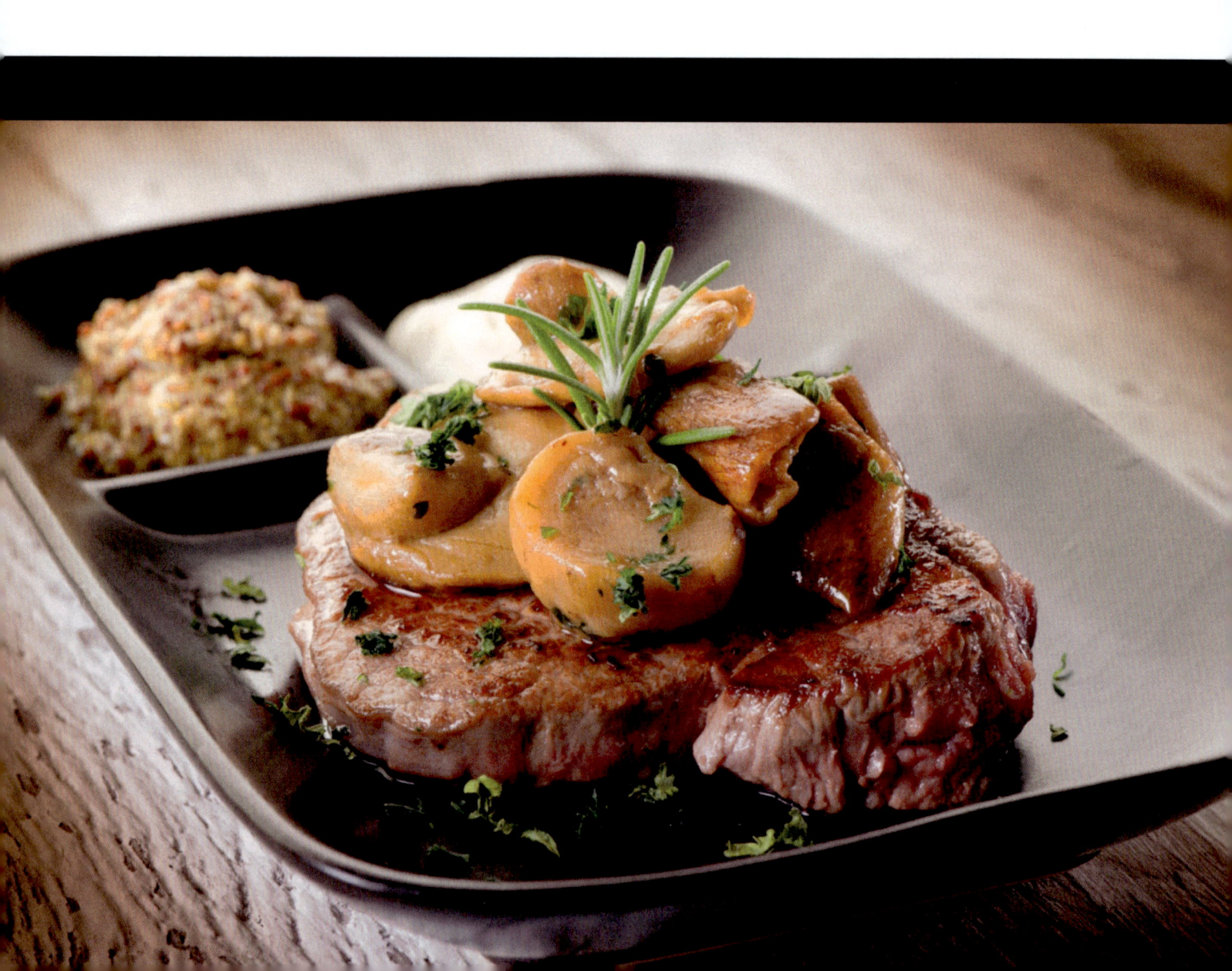

Directions

1. In 10-inch skillet, melt 1 tablespoon of the butter over medium-high heat. Sprinkle steaks with 1/2 teaspoon salt and 1/4 teaspoon pepper. Cook steaks 4 to 6 minutes, turning once, until deep brown. Reduce heat to low. Cover; cook 6 to 8 minutes for medium-rare to medium doneness (don't overcook; beef will continue to cook while standing). Remove beef to platter; cover to keep warm.

2. Increase heat to medium. Add remaining 2 tablespoons butter to skillet. Add mushrooms. Cook 3 to 4 minutes, stirring once or twice and scraping up any browned bits, until tender. Add wine and cooking sauce; heat to boiling. Reduce heat; simmer 3 to 5 minutes, stirring occasionally, until sauce is hot.

3. Serve mushroom sauce over steaks.

SANE Free Tools: SANESolution.com/Tools   Superfoods: store.SANESolution.com

SIRLOIN TIP ROAST

Total Time: 1hr 15 min
Prep: 15 min
Cook: 1hr

8 Servings
2 Nutrient-Dense Protein Per Serving
2 Whole-Food Fat Per Serving

Ingredients

- 1 tablespoon and 2 teaspoons paprika
- 1 tablespoon and 1 teaspoon kosher salt
- 1-1/4 teaspoons garlic powder
- 3/4 teaspoon ground black pepper
- 3/4 teaspoon onion powder
- 3/4 teaspoon ground cayenne pepper
- 3/4 teaspoon dried oregano
- 3/4 teaspoon dried thyme
- 2 tablespoons and 2 teaspoons extra virgin coconut oil
- 1-1/4 (3 pound) sirloin tip roast

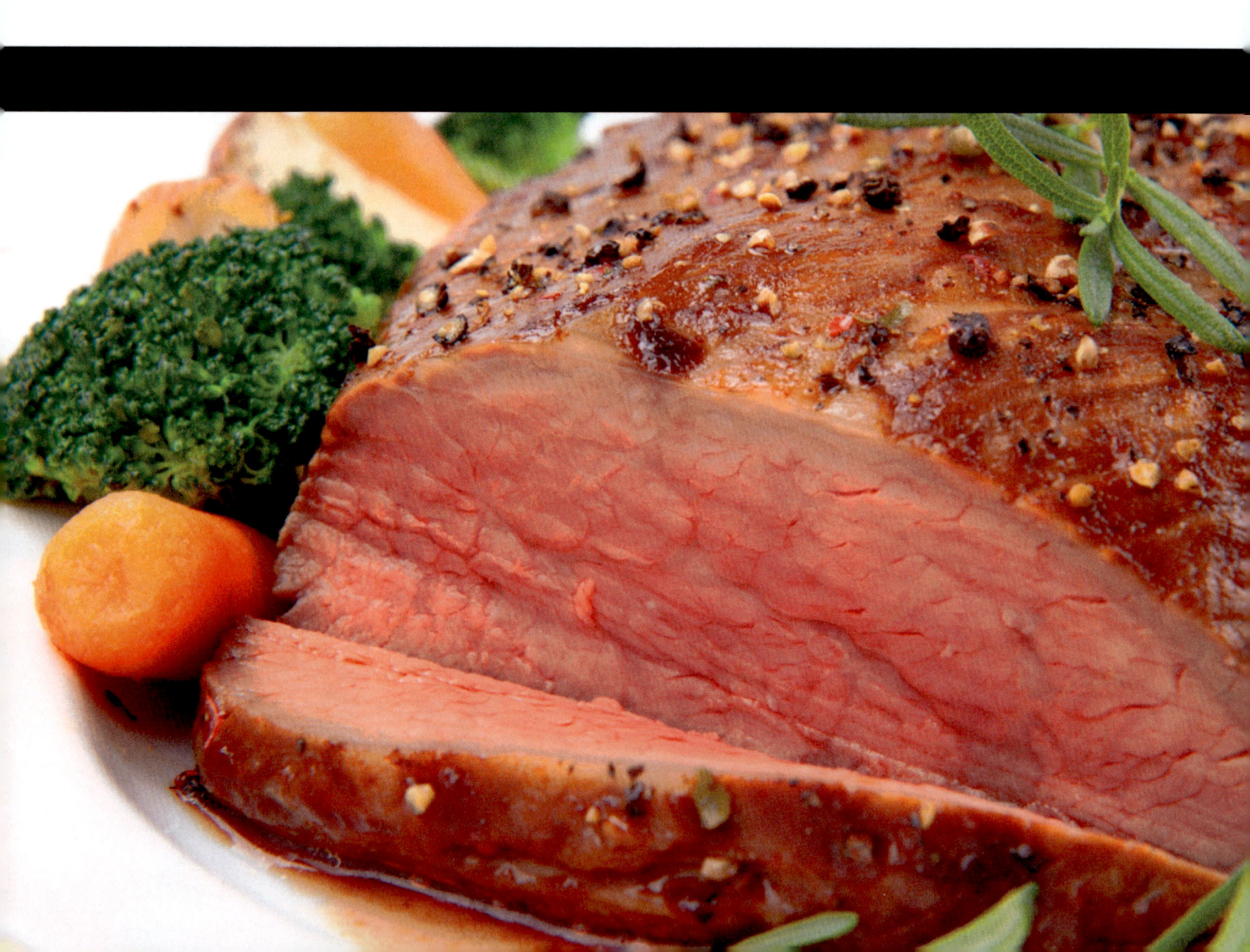

Directions

1. In a small bowl, mix the paprika, kosher salt, garlic powder, black pepper, onion powder, cayenne pepper, oregano, and thyme. Stir in melted extra virgin coconut oil, and allow the mixture to sit about 15 minutes.

2. Preheat oven to 350 degrees F (175 degrees C). Line a baking sheet with aluminum foil.

3. Place the roast on the prepared baking sheet, and cover on all sides with the spice mixture.

4. Roast 1 hour in the preheated oven, or to a minimum internal temperature of 145 degrees F (63 degrees C). Let sit 15 minutes before slicing.

Herb Garlic Beef Tenderloin

Total Time: 20 min
Prep: 10 min
Cook: 10 min

8 Servings
1 Nutrient-Dense Protein Per Serving
3 Whole-Food Fat Per Serving

Ingredients

- 5/8 (5 pound) whole beef tenderloin
- 3 tablespoons and 2 teaspoons extra virgin coconut oil
- 5 large garlic cloves, minced
- 1 tablespoon and 3/4 teaspoon minced fresh rosemary
- 1-3/4 teaspoons dried thyme leaves
- 1 tablespoon and 3/4 teaspoon coarsely ground black pepper
- 1-3/4 teaspoons salt

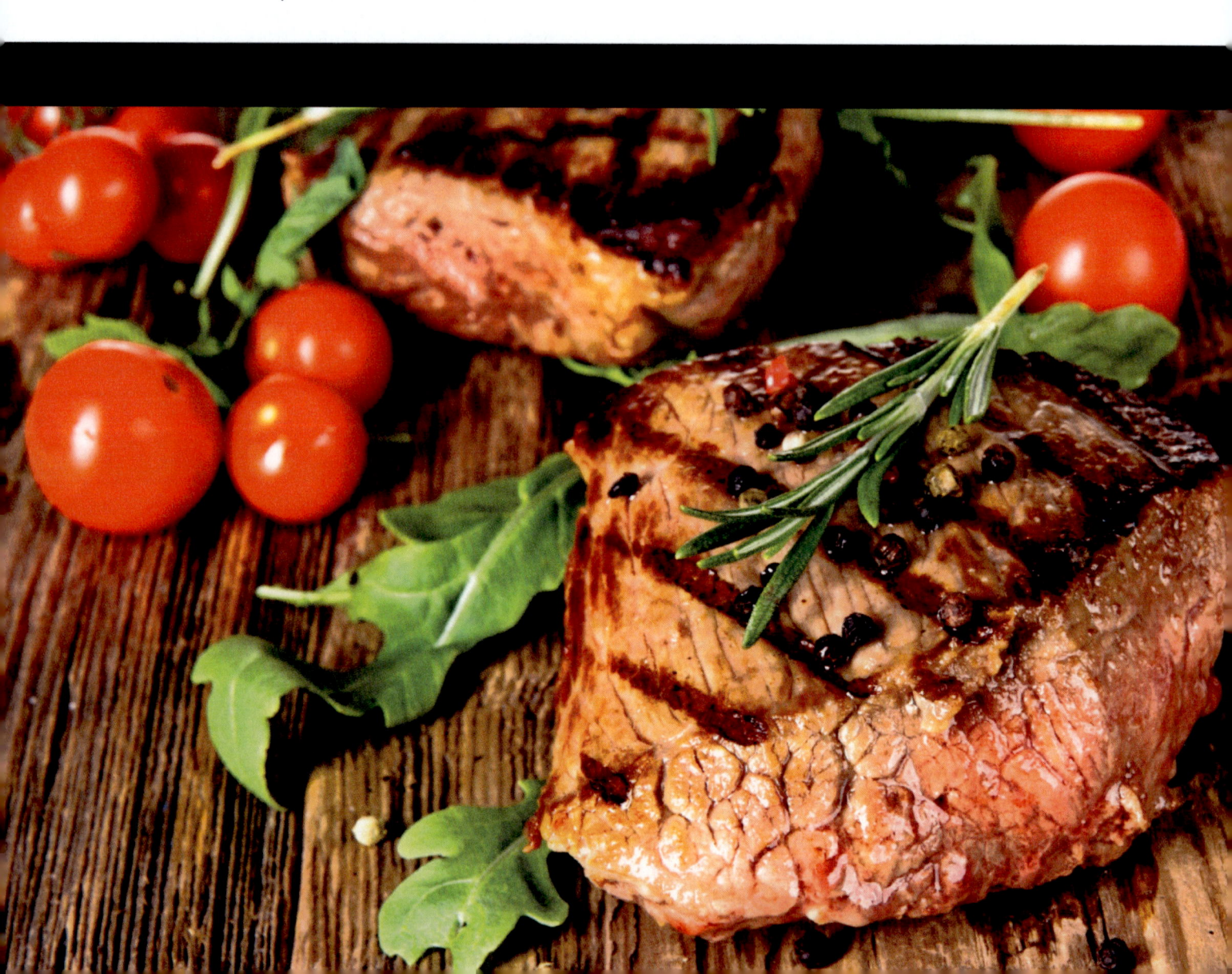

Directions

1. Prepare beef: Trim off excess fat with a sharp knife. Fold thin tip end under to approximate the thickness of the rest of the roast. Tie with butcher's twine, then keep tying the roast with twine every 11/2 to 2 inches (to help the roast keep its shape). Snip silverskin with scissors to keep roast from bowing during cooking. Then, mix oil, garlic, rosemary, thyme, pepper and salt; rub over roast to coat. Set meat aside.

2. Either build a charcoal fire in half the grill or turn all gas burners on high for 10 minutes. Lubricate grate with an oil-soaked rag using tongs. Place beef on hot rack and close lid; grill until well-seared, about 5 minutes. Turn meat and close lid; grill until well-seared on second side, another 5 minutes.

3. Move meat to the charcoal grill's cool side, or turn off burner directly underneath the meat and turn remaining one or two burners (depending on grill style) to medium. Cook until a meat thermometer inserted in the thickest section registers 130 degrees for rosy pink, 45 to 60 minutes, depending on tenderloin size and grill. Let meat rest 15 minutes before carving.

SANE   Free Tools: SANESolution.com/Tools   Superfoods: store.SANESolution.com

Tri Tip Roast

Total Time: 1hr 50 min
Prep: 10 min
Cook: 1hr 40 min

8 Servings
2 Nutrient-Dense Protein Per Serving
2 Whole-Food Fat Per Serving

Ingredients

- 1 tablespoon kosher salt
- 1 tablespoon finely ground black pepper
- 1 tablespoon granulated garlic
- 1 tablespoon onion powder
- 1 tablespoon dried oregano
- 1 teaspoon cayenne pepper
- 1 teaspoon dried rosemary
- 1/2 teaspoon dried sage
- 1/4 teaspoon lemon pepper
- 1/4 teaspoon seasoned salt
- 1/4 teaspoon beef bouillon granules
- 1 (3 pound) beef tri-tip roast

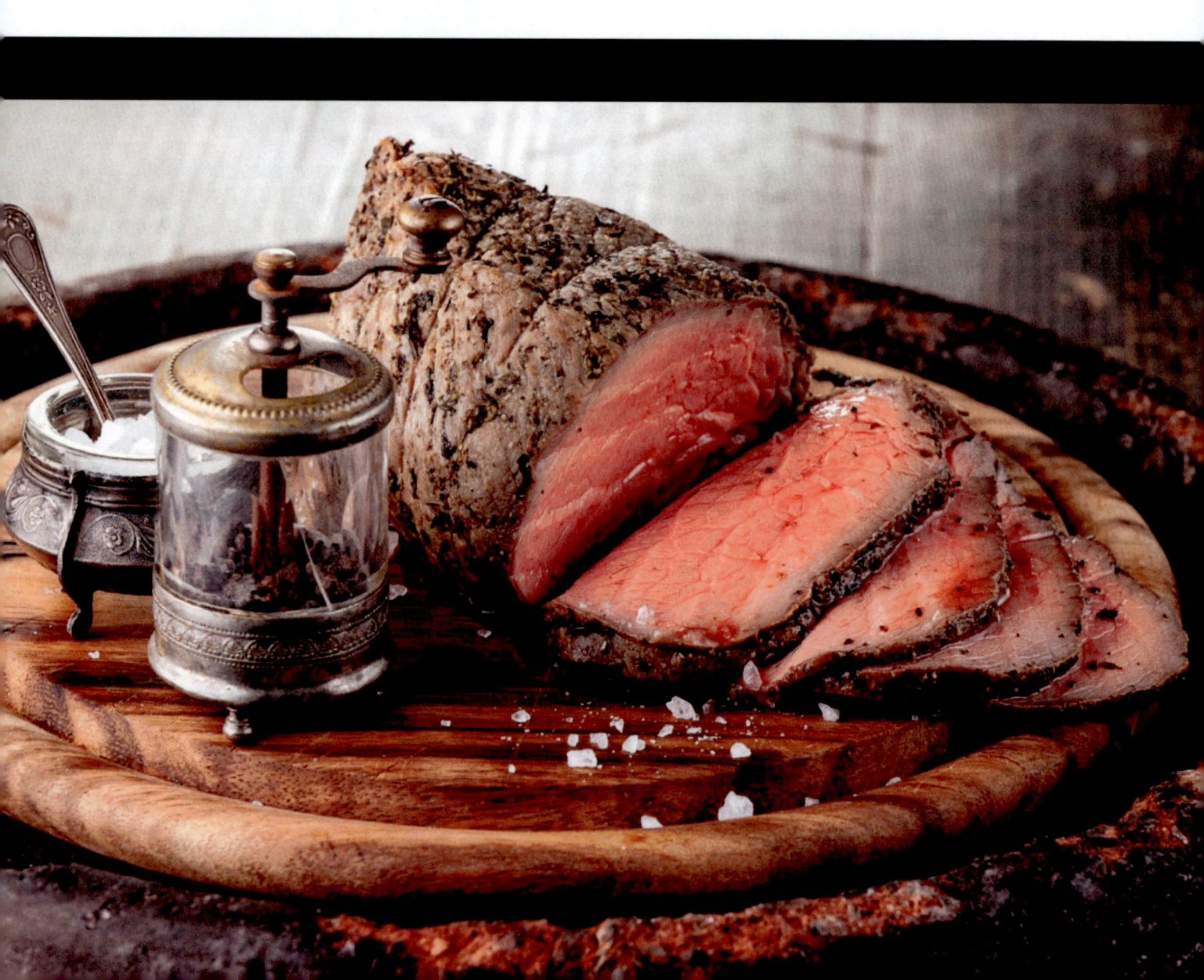

Directions

1. Preheat oven to 375 degrees F (190 degrees C).

2. Whisk kosher salt, black pepper, granulated garlic, onion powder, oregano, cayenne pepper, rosemary, sage, lemon pepper, seasoned salt, and beef bouillon together in a small bowl. Sprinkle spice mixture on all sides of roast and rub spices into meat.

3. Heat a skillet over high heat. Cook roast in hot skillet until browned, 2 to 3 minutes per side. Transfer meat, fat-side facing up, to a roasting pan. Cover the roasting pan with aluminum foil.

4. Roast in the preheated oven until just turning from pink to grey, about 90 minutes. An instant-read thermometer inserted into the center should read 150 degrees F (65 degrees C). Uncover roast and tent loosely with aluminum foil; let rest for 10 minutes before slicing across the grain.

Pork

Feta Pork

Total Time: 30 min
Prep: 10 min
Cook: 20 min

8 Servings
1 Nutrient-Dense Protein Per Serving
2 Whole-Food Fat Per Serving

Ingredients

- 2 teaspoons crushed dried rosemary
- 2 teaspoons dried basil
- 2 teaspoons minced garlic
- 2 pinches black pepper
- 1/4 cup extra virgin coconut oil
- 8 pork chops
- 2 cups fresh lemon juice
- 1 cup crumbled feta cheese with basil and sun-dried tomatoes

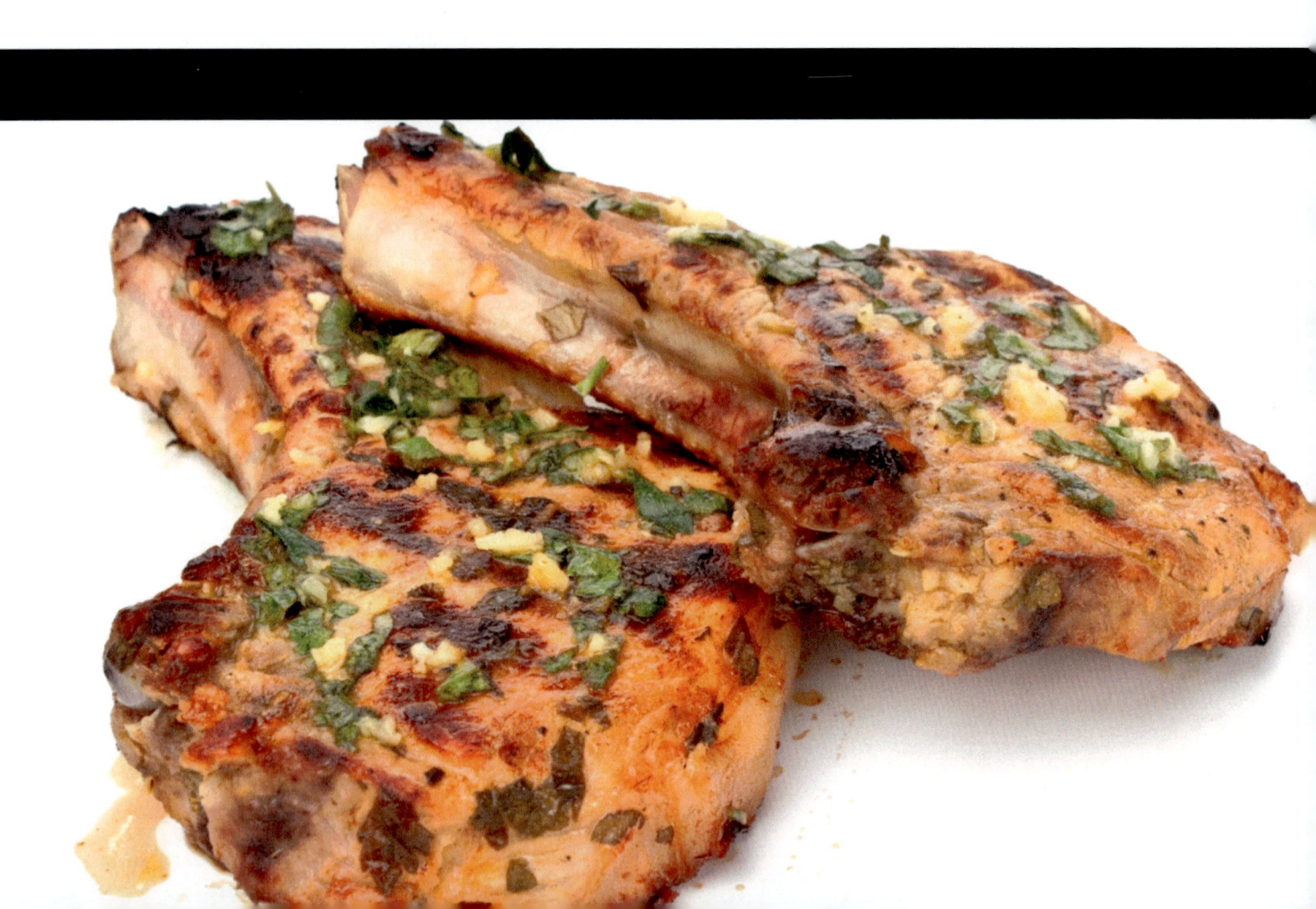

Directions

1. In a small bowl, stir together rosemary, basil, garlic, and pepper.

2. Heat extra virgin coconut oil in a large skillet over medium heat. Dip pork chops in lemon juice, and sprinkle both sides with herb mixture. Place pork chops in skillet, and sear both sides, about 7 minutes per side. Reduce heat to low. Sprinkle feta on top of chops; cover skillet, and cook until cheese begins to melt, about 5 minutes.

SANE Free Tools: SANESolution.com/Tools   Superfoods: store.SANESolution.com

Rosemary Pork Roast

Total Time: 2hr 20 min
Prep: 20 min
Cook: 2hr

8 Servings
2 Nutrient-Dense Protein Per Serving
1 Whole-Food Fat Per Serving

Ingredients

- 4 pounds pork tenderloin
- 1 tablespoon and 1 teaspoon extra virgin coconut oil
- 2-3/4 cloves garlic, minced
- 1/4 cup dried rosemary

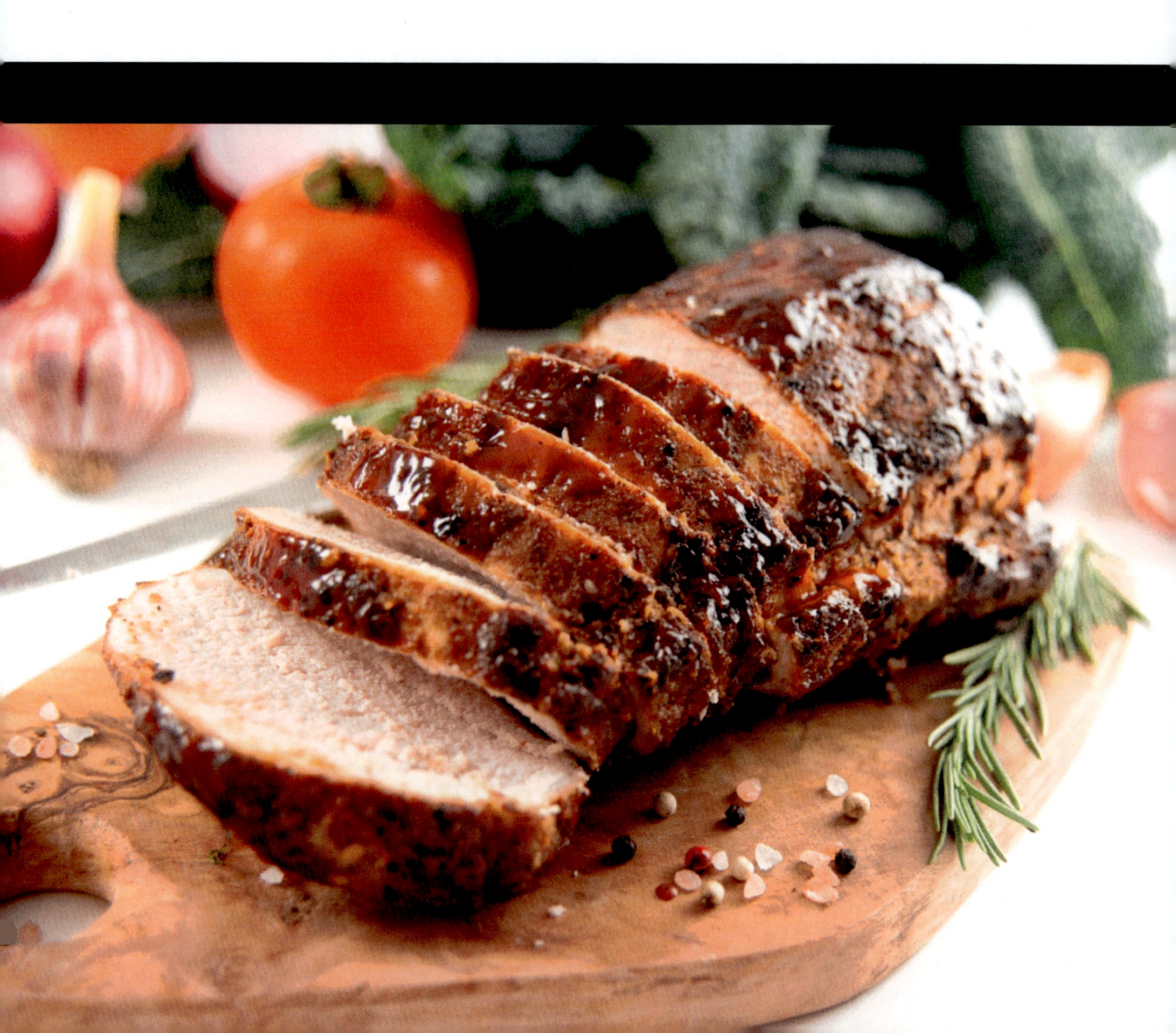

Directions

1. Preheat oven to 375 degrees F (190 degrees C).
2. Rub the roast OR tenderloin liberally with extra virgin coconut oil, then spread the garlic over it. Place it in a 10×15 inch roasting pan and sprinkle with the rosemary.
3. Bake at 375 degrees F (190 degrees C) for 2 hours, or until the internal temperature of the pork reaches 145 degrees F (63 degrees C).

SANE   Free Tools: SANESolution.com/Tools   Superfoods: store.SANESolution.com

Herbed Pork Chops

Total Time: 25 min
Prep: 10 min
Cook: 15 min

8 Servings
1 Nutrient-Dense Protein Per Serving
1 Whole-Food Fat Per Serving

Ingredients

- 1/3 cup lemon juice
- 2 tablespoons and 2 teaspoons extra virgin coconut oil
- 5-1/4 cloves garlic, minced
- 1-1/4 teaspoons salt
- 1/4 teaspoon dried oregano
- 1/4 teaspoon pepper
- 8 (4 ounce) boneless pork loin chops

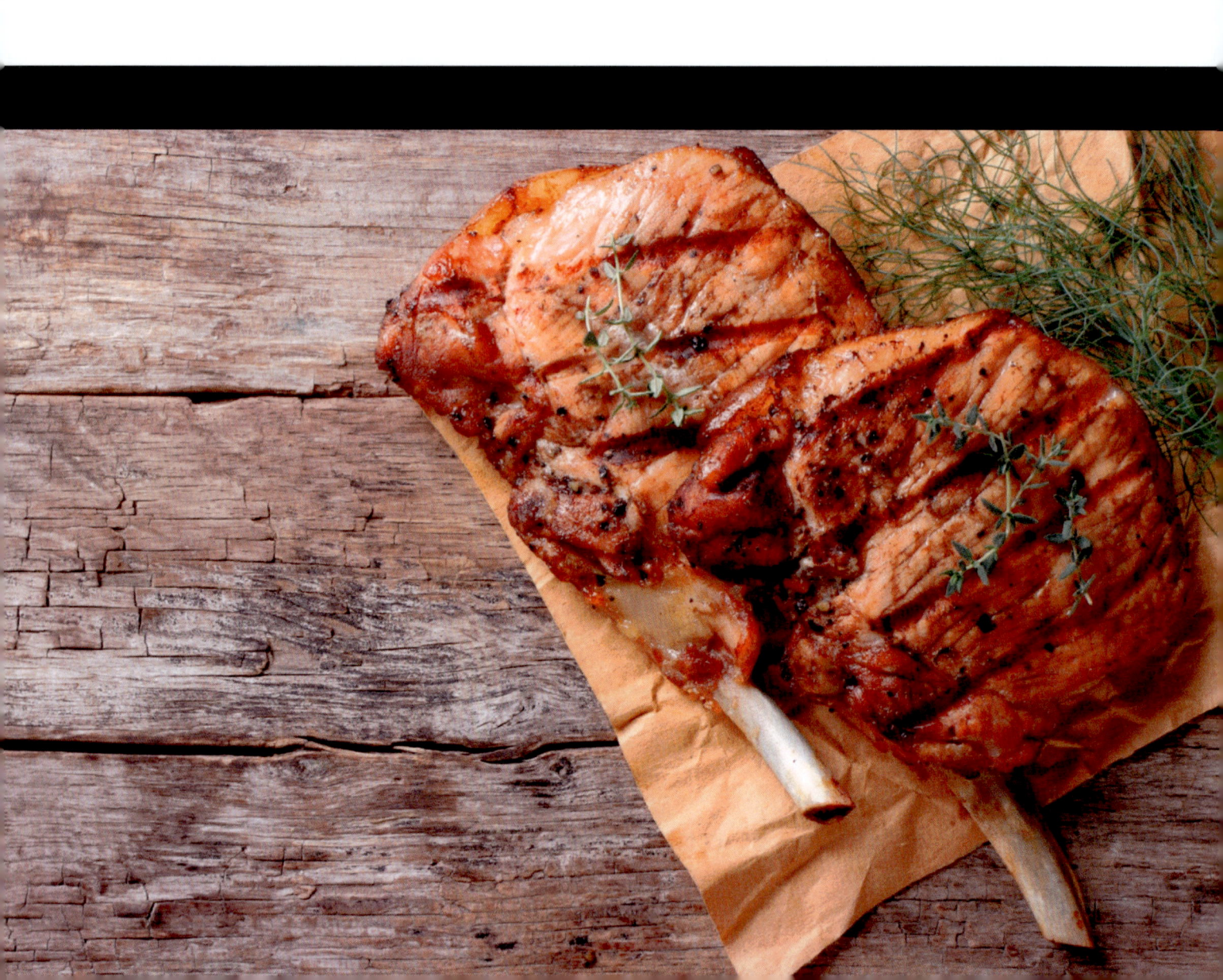

Directions

1. In a large resealable bag, combine lemon juice, melted oil, garlic, salt, oregano, and pepper. Place chops in bag, seal, and refrigerate 2 hours or overnight. Turn bag frequently to distribute marinade.

2. Preheat an outdoor grill for high heat. Remove chops from bag, and transfer remaining marinade to a saucepan. Bring marinade to a boil, remove from heat, and set aside.

3. Lightly oil the grill grate. Grill pork chops for 5 to 7 minutes per side, basting frequently with boiled marinade, until done.

SANE Free Tools: SANESolution.com/Tools   Superfoods: store.SANESolution.com

Grilled Pork Chops

Total Time: 35 min
Prep: 10 min
Cook: 25 min

8 Servings
1 Nutrient-Dense Protein Per Serving
2 Whole-Food Fat Per Serving

Ingredients

- 2 tablespoons seasoned salt
- 2 teaspoons ground black pepper
- 2 tablespoons garlic powder
- 2 tablespoons onion powder
- 2 tablespoons ground paprika
- 1 tablespoon and 1 teaspoon Worcestershire sauce
- 2 teaspoons liquid smoke flavoring
- 8 bone-in pork chops (1/2 to 3/4 inch thick)

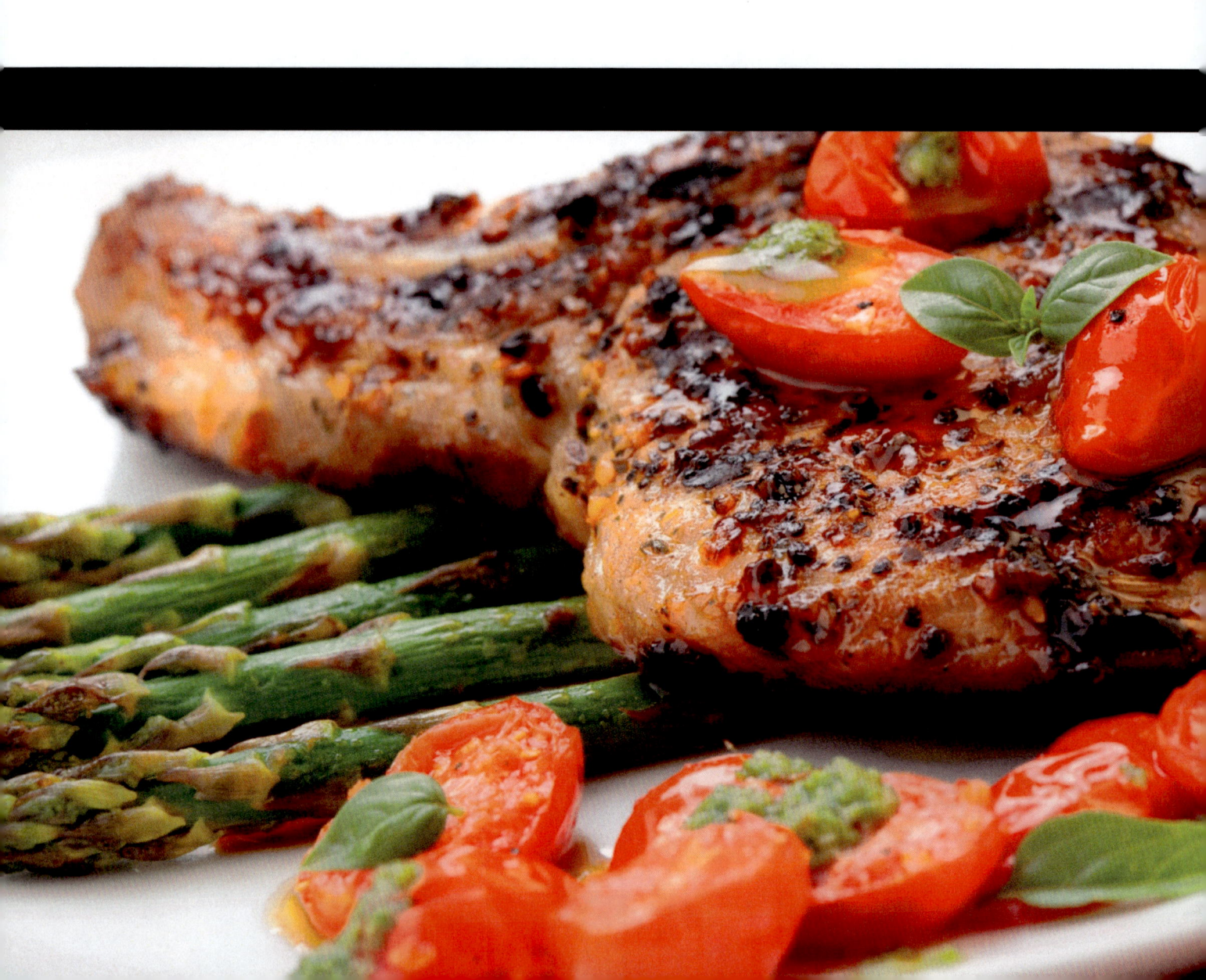

Directions

1. Preheat an outdoor grill for medium heat, and lightly oil the grate.

2. In a bowl, mix together the seasoned salt, black pepper, garlic powder, onion powder, paprika, Worcestershire sauce, and smoke flavoring until thoroughly combined. Rinse pork chops, and sprinkle the wet chops on both sides with the spice mixture. With your hands, massage the spice rub into the meat; allow to stand for 10 minutes.

3. Grill the chops over indirect heat until no longer pink inside, about 12 minutes per side. An instant-read thermometer should read at least 145 degrees F (63 degrees C). Allow chops to stand for 10 more minutes before serving.

SANE   Free Tools: SANESolution.com/Tools   Superfoods: store.SANESolution.com

Pork Burgundy

Total Time: 1hr 30 min
Prep: 30 min
Cook: 1hr

8 Servings
2 Nutrient-Dense Protein Per Serving
1 Whole-Food Fat Per Serving

Ingredients

- 4 pounds pork tenderloin
- 1 teaspoon salt
- 1 teaspoon ground black pepper
- 1 teaspoon garlic powder
- 1 onion, thinly sliced
- 2 stalks celery, chopped
- 4 cups red wine
- 2 (.75 ounce) packets dry brown gravy mix

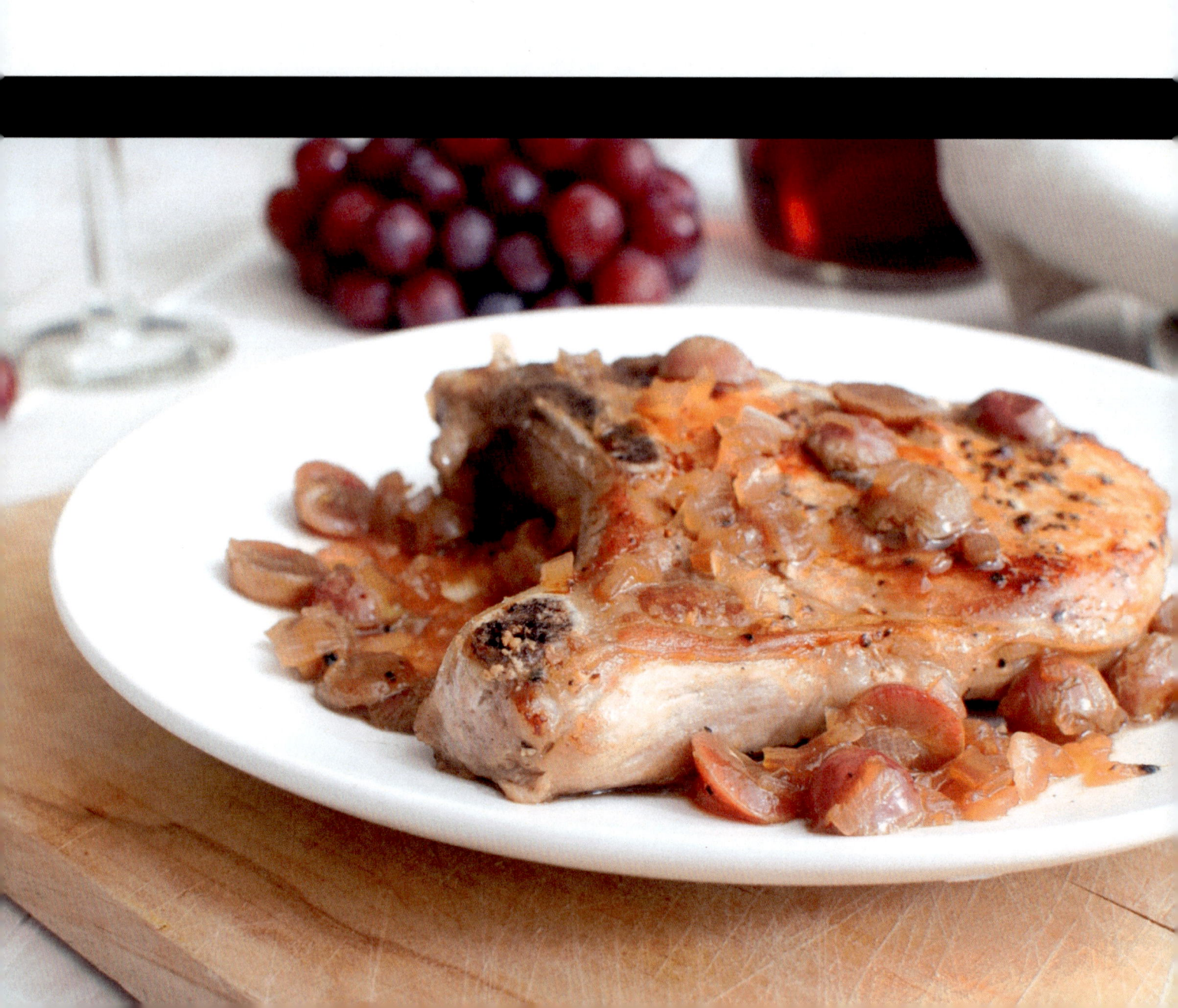

Directions

1. Preheat oven to 350 degrees F (175 degrees C).

2. Place pork in a 9×13 inch baking dish, and sprinkle meat with salt, pepper and garlic powder. Top with onion and celery, and pour wine over all.

3. Bake in the preheated oven for 45 minutes.

4. When done baking, remove meat from baking dish, and place on a serving platter. Pour gravy mix into baking dish with wine and cooking juices, and stir until thickened. Slice meat, and cover with the gravy.

SANE   Free Tools: SANESolution.com/Tools   Superfoods: store.SANESolution.com

Italian Pork Chops

Total Time: 1hr 25 min
Prep: 15 min
Cook: 1hr 10 min

8 Servings
2 Nutrient-Dense Protein Per Serving
1 Whole-Food Fat Per Serving

Ingredients

- 1-1/4 teaspoons extra virgin coconut oil
- 2 tablespoons and 2 teaspoons extra virgin coconut oil
- 2-2/3 cups sliced mushrooms
- 8 (3/4 inch thick) pork loin chops
- 2-3/4 cloves garlic, crushed
- 1-1/3 cups chopped onion
- 1-1/4 (14.5 ounce) cans diced Italian tomatoes, undrained
- 1-1/4 teaspoons dried basil
- 3/4 teaspoon dried oregano
- 3/4 teaspoon salt
- 1/4 teaspoon ground black pepper
- 2/3 cup water, if necessary
- 1-1/4 large green bell pepper, cut in 6 pieces

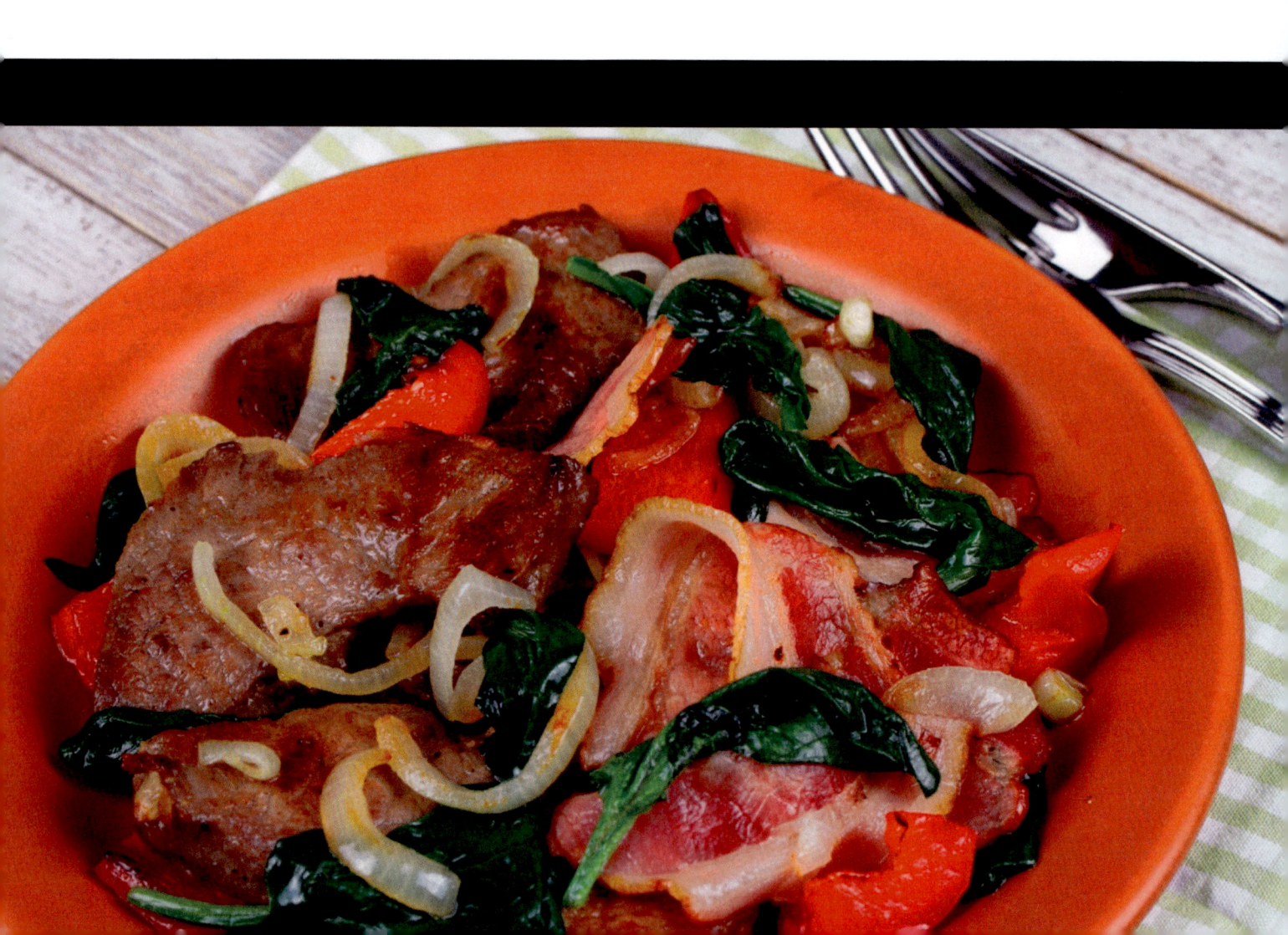

Directions

1. Heat 1 teaspoon extra virgin coconut oil in a skillet over medium heat. Stir in mushrooms; cook and stir until mushrooms are tender, 5 to 7 minutes. Transfer the mushrooms to a bowl and set aside.

2. Heat the remaining 2 tablespoons extra virgin coconut oil in the skillet over medium heat. Add the pork chops, browning on both sides, 7 to 10 minutes. Place the pork chops on a plate, then drain all but 1 tablespoon of drippings from the skillet. Stir in the garlic and onion; cook and stir until the onion has softened and turned translucent, about 5 minutes.

3. Pour in the tomatoes, then season with basil, oregano, salt, and pepper. Transfer the pork chops back to the skillet; cover and simmer until the pork chops are tender and no longer pink in the center, about 45 minutes. Stir in some water if the mixture becomes too dry. Place the bell pepper on top of the pork, then add the reserved mushrooms. Continue to simmer until the bell pepper is tender, 5 to 10 minutes.

SANE   Free Tools: SANESolution.com/Tools   Superfoods: store.SANESolution.com

Mustard Soy Tenderloin

Total Time: 1hr 15 min
Prep: 15 min
Cook: 1hr

8 Servings
1 Nutrient-Dense Protein Per Serving
2 Whole-Food Fat Per Serving

Ingredients

- 1/3 cup red wine
- 1/3 cup soy sauce
- 2 tablespoons light brown sugar
- 2 pounds pork tenderloin
- 1/3 cup all-natural mayonnaise
- 1/3 cup sour cream
- 1 1/2 tablespoons mustard powder
- 1 tablespoon minced fresh chives (optional)

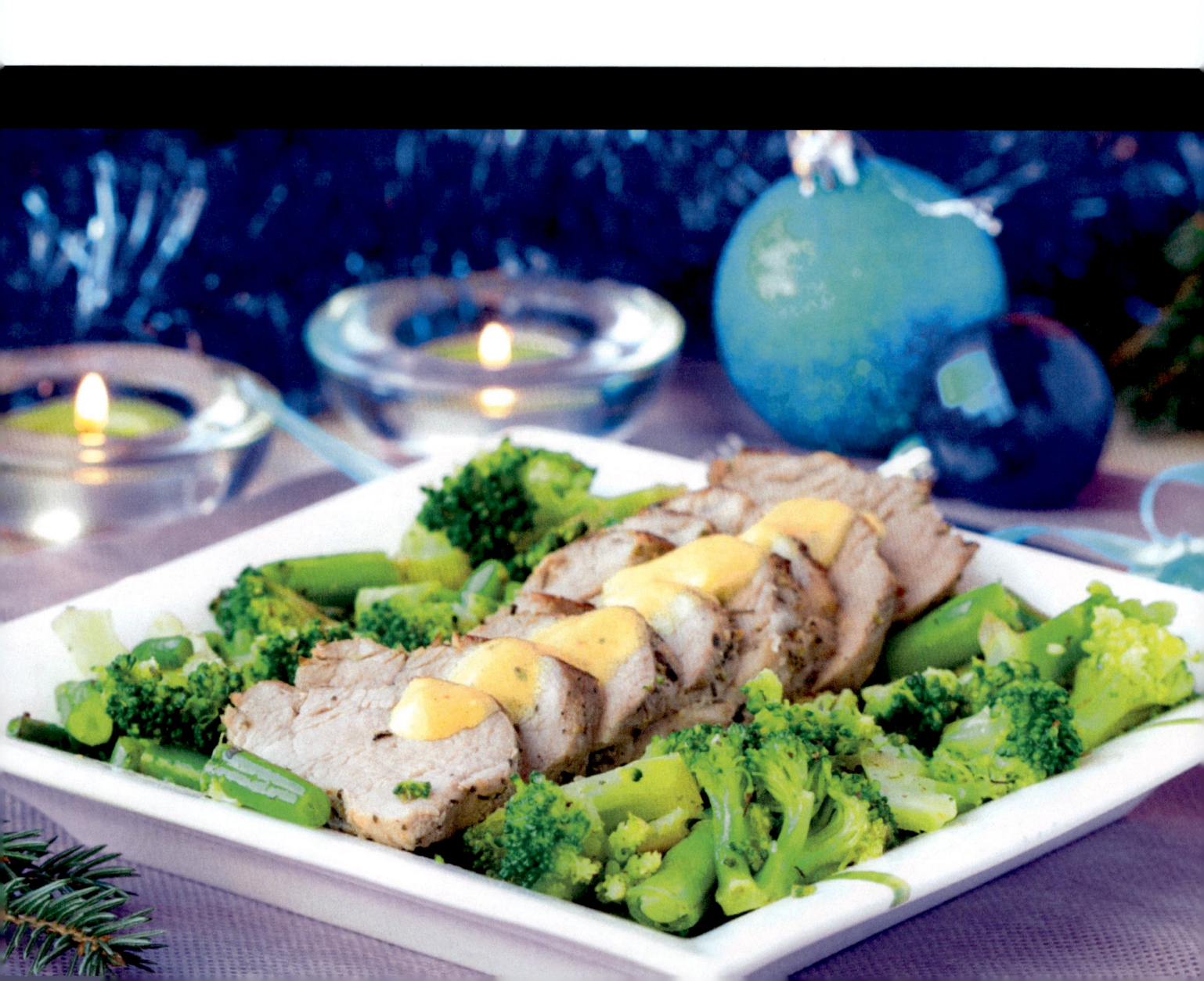

Directions

1. Combine wine, soy sauce, and brown sugar in a large resealable plastic bag. Place tenderloin in bag, and refrigerate overnight, or at least 8 hours.

2. In a small bowl, combine mayonnaise, sour cream, mustard powder; mix well. Mix in minced chives if you wish. Chill until ready to serve.

3. Preheat oven to 325 degrees F (165 degrees C). Place meat and marinade in a shallow baking dish, and roast for 1 hour, basting occasionally. Temperature of meat should register 145 degrees F (63 degrees C). Let rest for a few minutes, then cut into 1/2 inch thick slices. Serve with mustard sauce.

SANE Free Tools: SANESolution.com/Tools   Superfoods: store.SANESolution.com

White Wine Pork Chops

Total Time: 25 min
Prep: 10 min
Cook: 15 min

8 Servings
1 Nutrient-Dense Protein Per Serving
3 Whole-Food Fat Per Serving

Ingredients

- 3 tablespoons butter
- 8 boneless pork chops
- salt, to taste
- ground black pepper, to taste
- 3/4 cup white wine
- 3/4 cup heavy cream
- 1 (8 ounce) package sliced fresh mushrooms

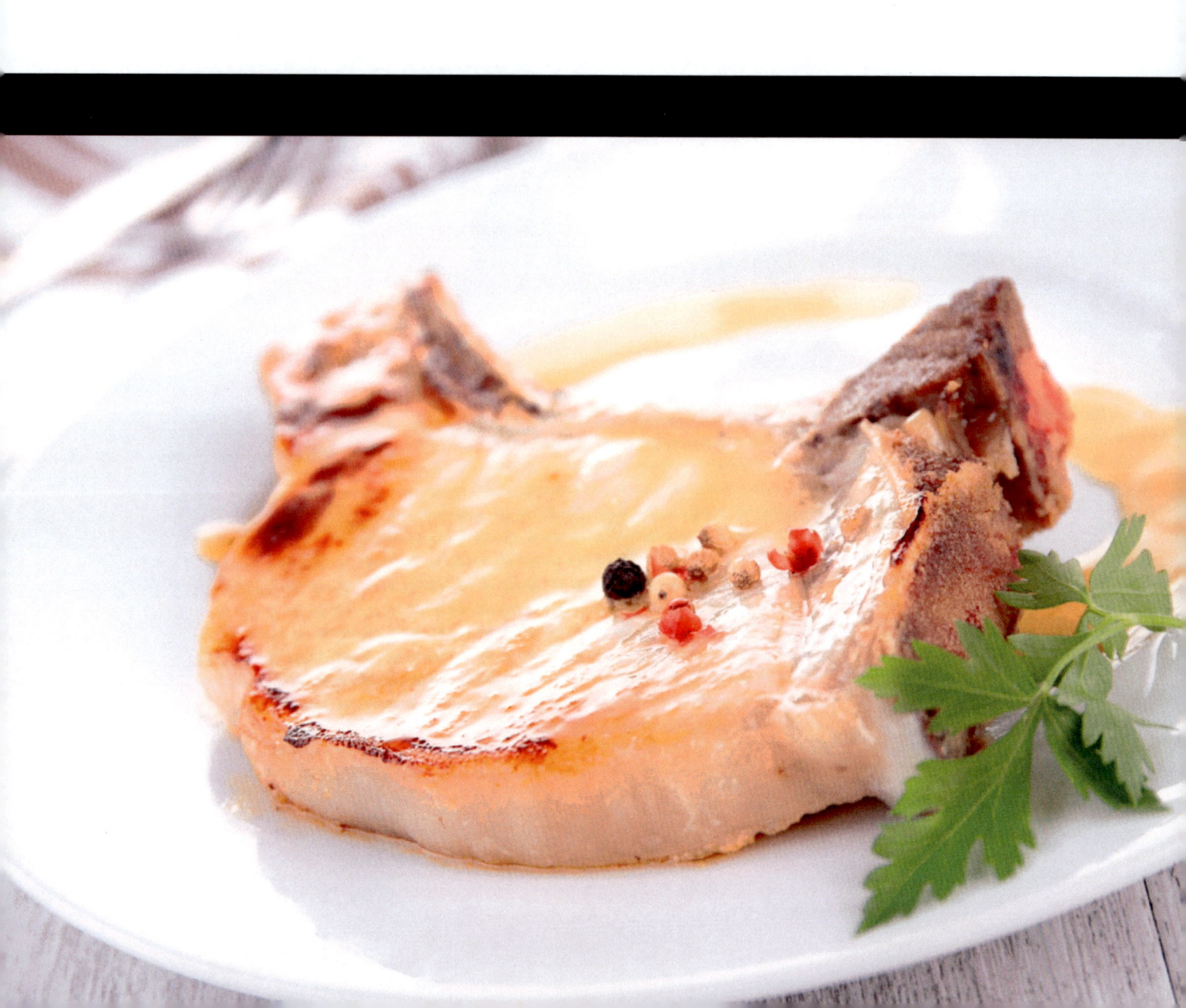

Directions

1. Melt butter in a large skillet over medium heat. Season pork chops with salt and pepper, and arrange in a single layer in pan. Pan-fry for 2 minutes on each side to brown. Pour in wine, and continue cooking for 6 minutes. Remove chops from pan.

2. Pour cream into the skillet, and then add mushrooms. Increase heat to high; cook for 5 minutes, stirring frequently, until sauce reduces and thickens. Return chops to pan to warm before serving.

Stuffed Pork Chops

Total Time: 35 min
Prep: 15 min
Cook: 20 min

8 Servings
2 Nutrient-Dense Protein Per Serving
3 Whole-Food Fat Per Serving
1 Most Dairy Per Serving

Ingredients

- 8 boneless pork loin chops, butterflied
- 1 pound crumbled blue cheese
- 8 slices bacon – cooked and crumbled
- 1/2 cup chopped fresh chives
- garlic salt to taste
- ground black pepper to taste
- chopped fresh parsley for garnish

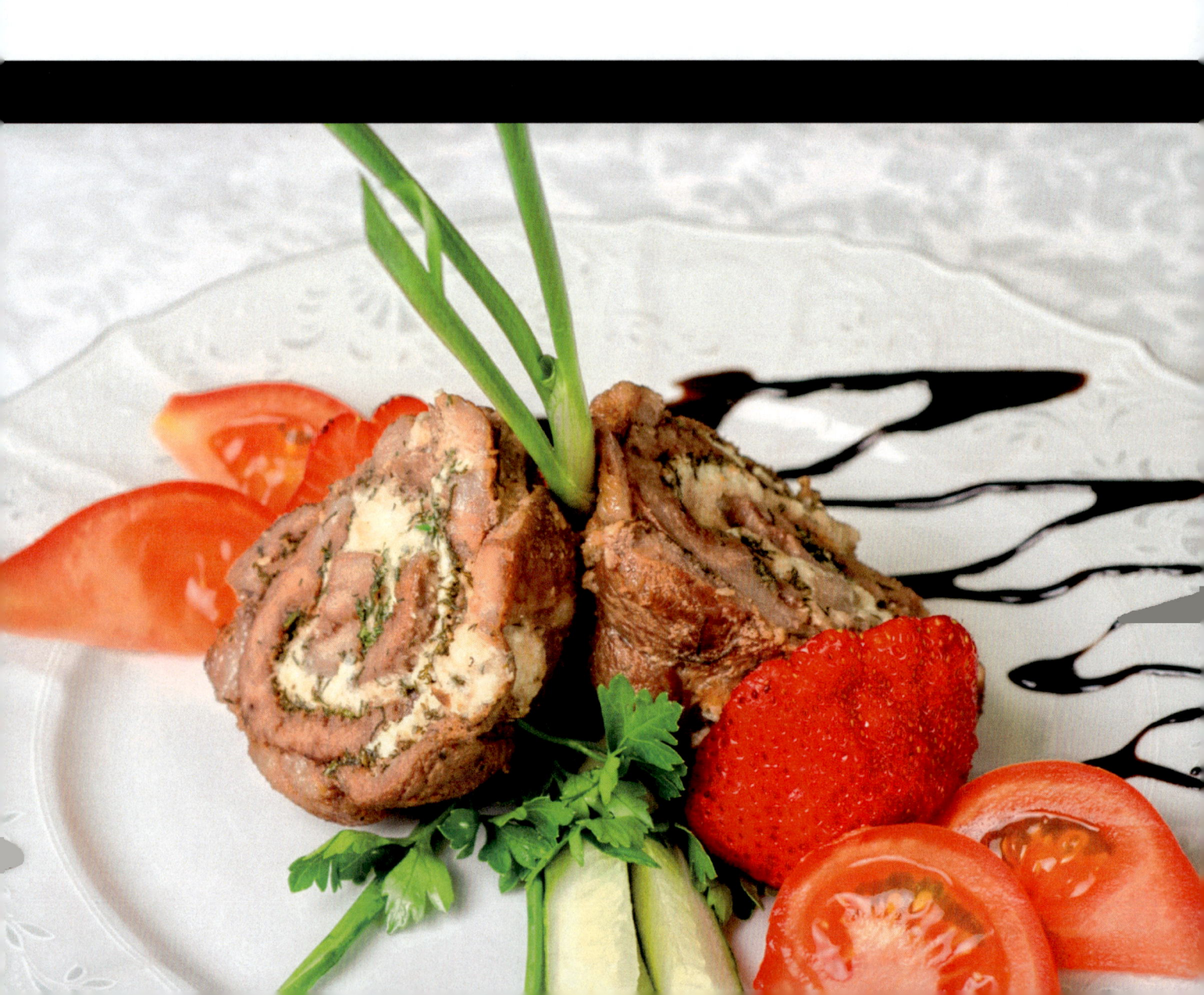

Directions

1. Preheat the oven to 325 degrees F (165 degrees C). Grease a shallow baking dish.

2. In a small bowl, mix together the blue cheese, bacon and chives. Divide into halves, and pack each half into a loose ball. Place each one into a pocket of a butterflied pork chop, close, and secure with toothpicks. Season each chop with garlic salt and pepper. Keep in mind that the blue cheese will be salty. Place in the prepared baking dish.

3. Bake for 20 minutes in the preheated oven, or it may take longer if your chops are thicker. Cook until the stuffing is hot, and chops are to your desired degree of doneness. Garnish with fresh parsley and serve.

South American Roast Pork

Total Time: 2hr 40 min
Prep: 10 min
Cook: 2hr 30 min

8 Servings
2 Nutrient-Dense Protein Per Serving
2 Whole-Food Fat Per Serving
1 Most Dairy Per Serving

Ingredients

- 4 cloves garlic
- 2 teaspoons kosher salt
- 1 teaspoon ground black pepper
- 1 teaspoon ground cumin
- 1 teaspoon dried oregano
- 1 teaspoon ground coriander
- 3 tablespoons lime juice
- 3 tablespoons orange juice
- 3 tablespoons extra virgin coconut oil
- 1 1/2 teaspoons white wine vinegar
- 1 (4 pound) pork shoulder roast

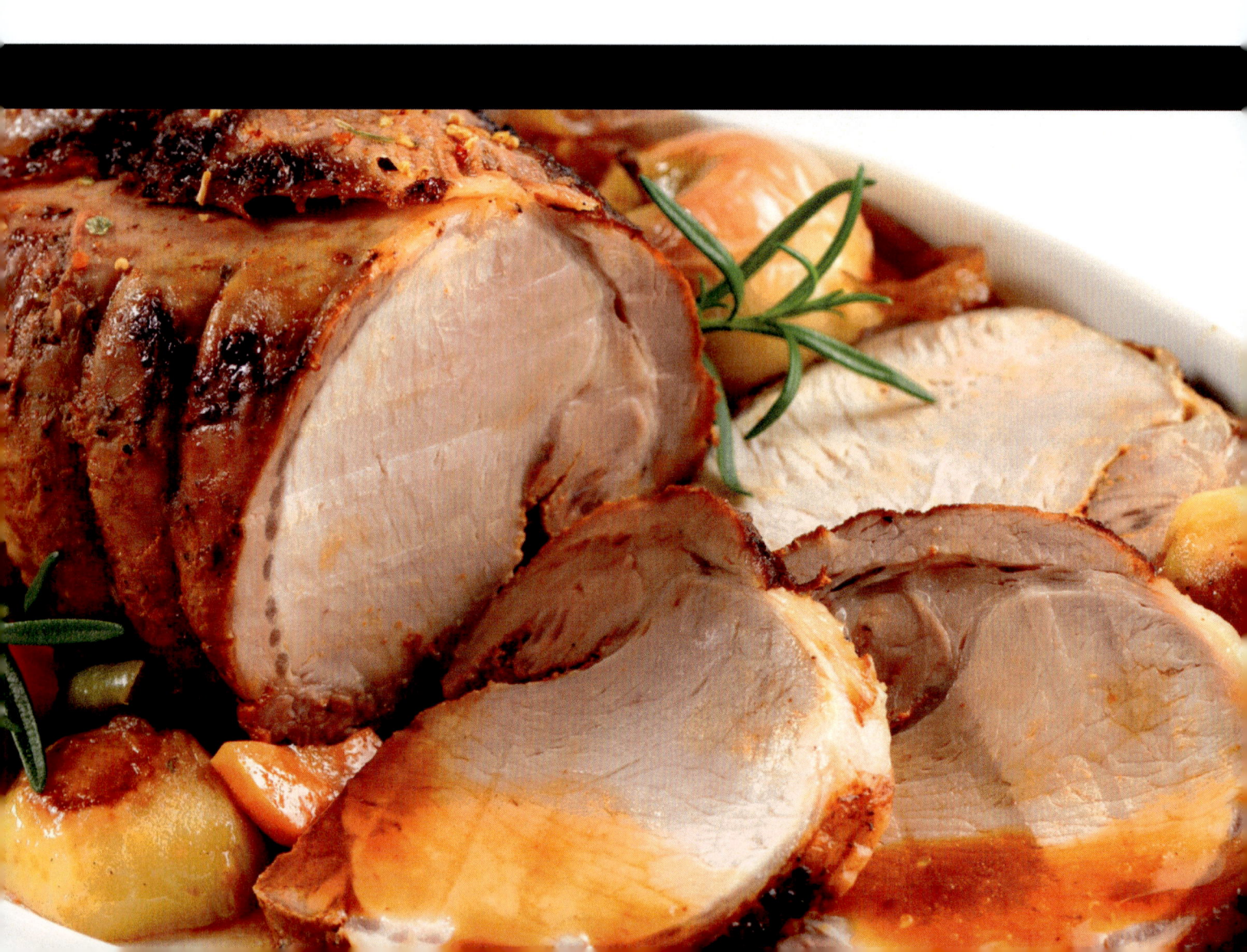

Directions

1. Grind garlic, salt, black pepper, cumin, oregano, and coriander into a paste using a mortar and pestle.

2. Transfer half of the garlic and spice paste to a bowl; add lime juice, orange juice, melted coconut oil, and vinegar. Beat the mixture with a whisk until smooth.

3. Cut several inch-long, deep slits into the fatty side of the pork roast. Rub the reserved garlic paste into the slits.

4. Put rubbed roast into a gallon-size resealable plastic bag. Pour the liquid mixture over the roast, squeeze as much air from the bag as possible and seal; refrigerate, turning occasionally, 8 hours to overnight.

5. Remove pork roast from refrigerator, put into a roasting pan, and let warm at room temperature for 30 minutes.

6. Preheat oven to 400 degrees F (200 degrees C).

7. Roast pork in preheated oven for 30 minutes, reduce heat to 375 degrees F (190 degrees C), and continue cooking until pork is no longer pink in the center, about 2 hours more. An instant-read thermometer inserted into the center should read at least 170 degrees F (75 degrees C).

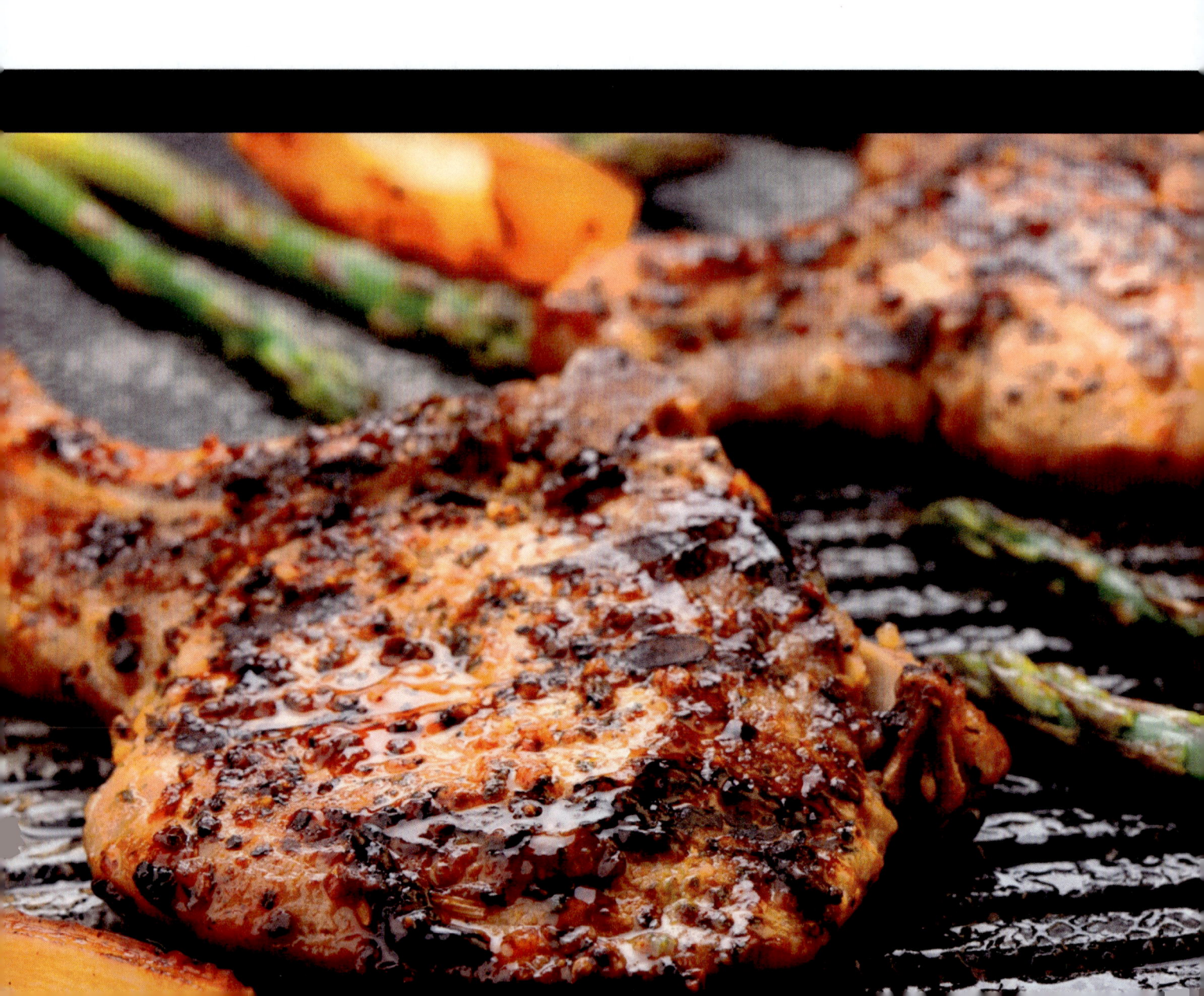

SANE

Free Tools: SANESolution.com/Tools   Superfoods: store.SANESolution.com

Chili Chops

Total Time: 30 min
Prep: 10 min
Cook: 20 min

8 Servings
1 Nutrient-Dense Protein Per Serving
1 Whole-Food Fat Per Serving

Ingredients

- 3/4 cup soy sauce
- 1/4 cup fresh lemon juice
- 1 tablespoon brown sugar
- 1 tablespoon chili sauce
- 1/4 teaspoon garlic powder
- 8 center cut pork chops

Directions

1. In a large resealable bag, mix together the soy sauce, lemon juice, brown sugar, chili sauce, and garlic powder.. Place the pork chops into the bag, carefully seal the bag, and marinate for 6-12 hours in the refrigerator. Turn the bag over about halfway through.

2. Preheat an outdoor grill for high heat.

3. Arrange pork chops on the lightly oiled grate, and cook 5 to 7 minutes on each side, until the internal temperature reaches 145 degrees F (63 degrees C).

SEAFOOD

TIP: Not familiar with the SANE Food Group or SANE Serving Sizes?

It's all good! Get everything you need by attending your FREE masterclass at SANESeminar.com and by downloading your FREE tools at SANESolution.com/Tools.

SANE   Free Tools: SANESolution.com/Tools   Superfoods: store.SANESolution.com

Cod

Lemon Pepper Cod

Total Time: 15 min
Prep: 5 min
Cook: 10 min

8 Servings
1 Nutrient-Dense Protein Per Serving
1 Whole-Food Fat Per Serving

Ingredients

- 1/4 cup and 2 tablespoons extra virgin coconut oil
- 3 pounds cod fillets
- 2 lemon, juiced
- ground black pepper to taste

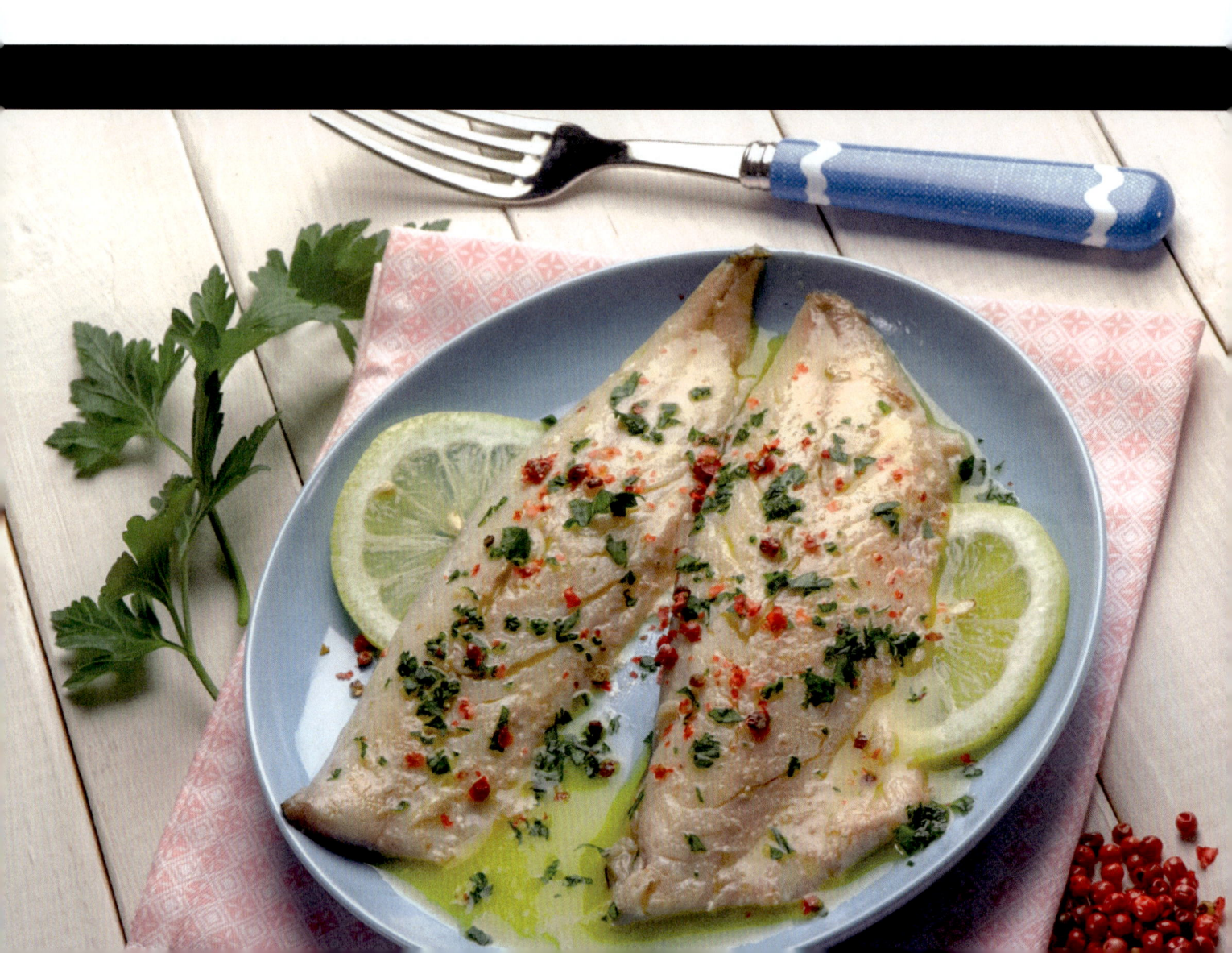

Directions

1. In a large skillet, heat oil over medium high heat until hot. Add fillets and squeeze 1/2 of the lemon's juice over the tops. Sprinkle with pepper to taste. Cook for 4 minutes and turn. Squeeze with the remaining lemon's juice and sprinkle with pepper to taste. Continue to cook until fillets flake easily with a fork.

Spinach and Tomatoes Cod

Total Time: 20 min
Prep: 10 min
Cook: 10 min

8 Servings
1 Nutrient-Dense Protein Per Serving
2 Whole-Food Fat Per Serving

Ingredients

- 8 (4 ounce) fillets cod
- salt and ground black pepper to taste
- 8 pinches garlic powder, or to taste
- 2 cups roughly chopped spinach, or to taste
- 2 tomato, seeded and diced
- 1/2 cup chopped onion
- 1/2 cup extra virgin coconut oil, or to taste
- 1/2 cup balsamic vinegar, or to taste
- 8 slices mozzarella cheese, cut into cubes

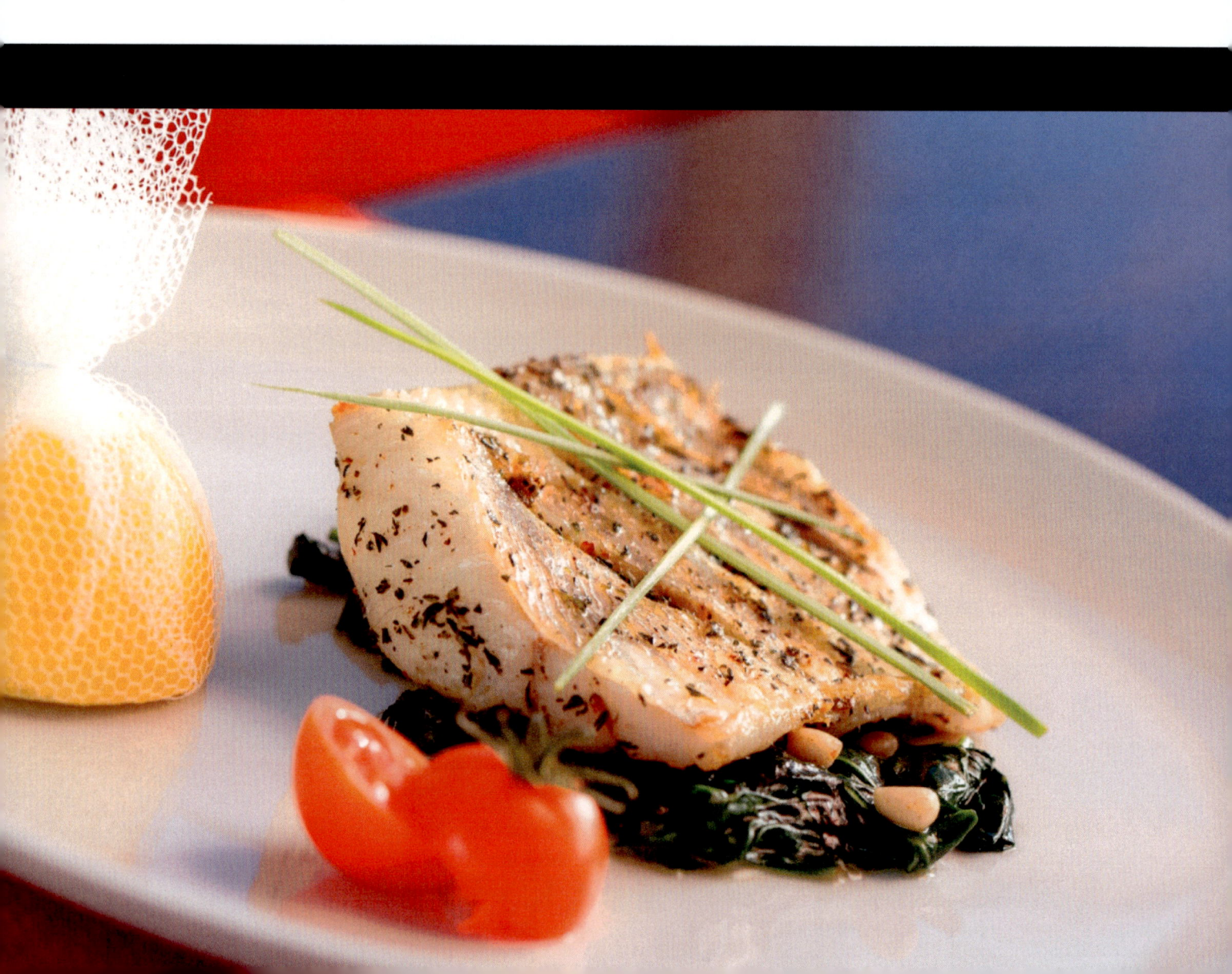

Directions

1. Preheat an outdoor grill for medium-high heat.

2. Place cod on a piece of aluminum foil and season with salt, black pepper, and garlic powder. Top cod with spinach, tomato, and onion; season again with salt and black pepper. Drizzle extra virgin coconut oil and balsamic vinegar over cod and top with mozzarella cheese. Fold foil over cod creating a packet, crimping the edges together making a seal.

3. Cook on the preheated grill until fish flakes easily with a fork, 7 to 9 minutes.

SANE Free Tools: SANESolution.com/Tools   Superfoods: store.SANESolution.com

Bacon Wrapped Cod

Total Time: 25 min
Prep: 15 min
Cook: 10 min

8 Servings
2 Nutrient-Dense Protein Per Serving
1 Whole-Food Fat Per Serving

Ingredients

- 8 (6 ounce) fillets cod
- 2 tablespoons extra virgin coconut oil
- 2 tablespoons chili sauce
- 8 slices bacon
- 1 leek, chopped
- 1 ounce enoki mushrooms

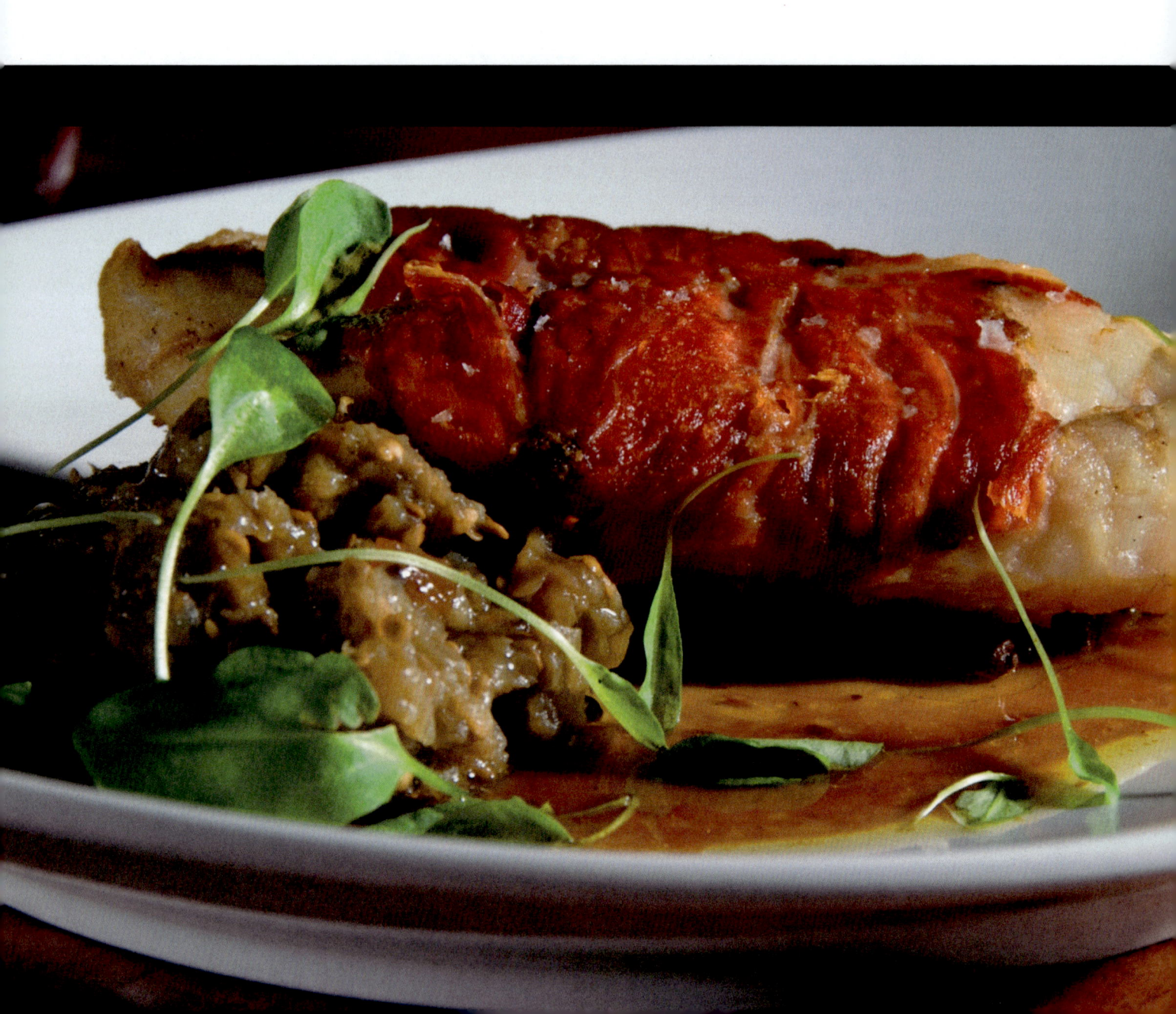

Directions

1. Preheat an outdoor grill for high heat. Soak some toothpicks in water while the grill heats up.

2. Spread a thin layer of melted extra virgin coconut oil and chili sauce onto one side of each fish fillet. At one end, place some of the leek and a couple of mushrooms. Roll towards the other end. Wrap each roll with a slice of bacon, and secure with two toothpicks.

3. Place on the preheated grill, and cook covered for 5 minutes. Be careful of flare-ups from the bacon grease. Turn over, and cook for 5 more minutes, until bacon is crisp and fish flakes easily.

SANE   Free Tools: SANESolution.com/Tools   Superfoods: store.SANESolution.com

Sesame Cod

Total Time: 15 min
Prep: 5 min
Cook: 10 min

8 Servings
2 Nutrient-Dense Protein Per Serving
1 Whole-Food Fat Per Serving

Ingredients

- 3 pounds cod fillets
- 2 teaspoons butter, melted
- 2 teaspoons lemon juice
- 2 teaspoons dried tarragon
- 2 pinches ground black pepper
- 2 tablespoons sesame seeds

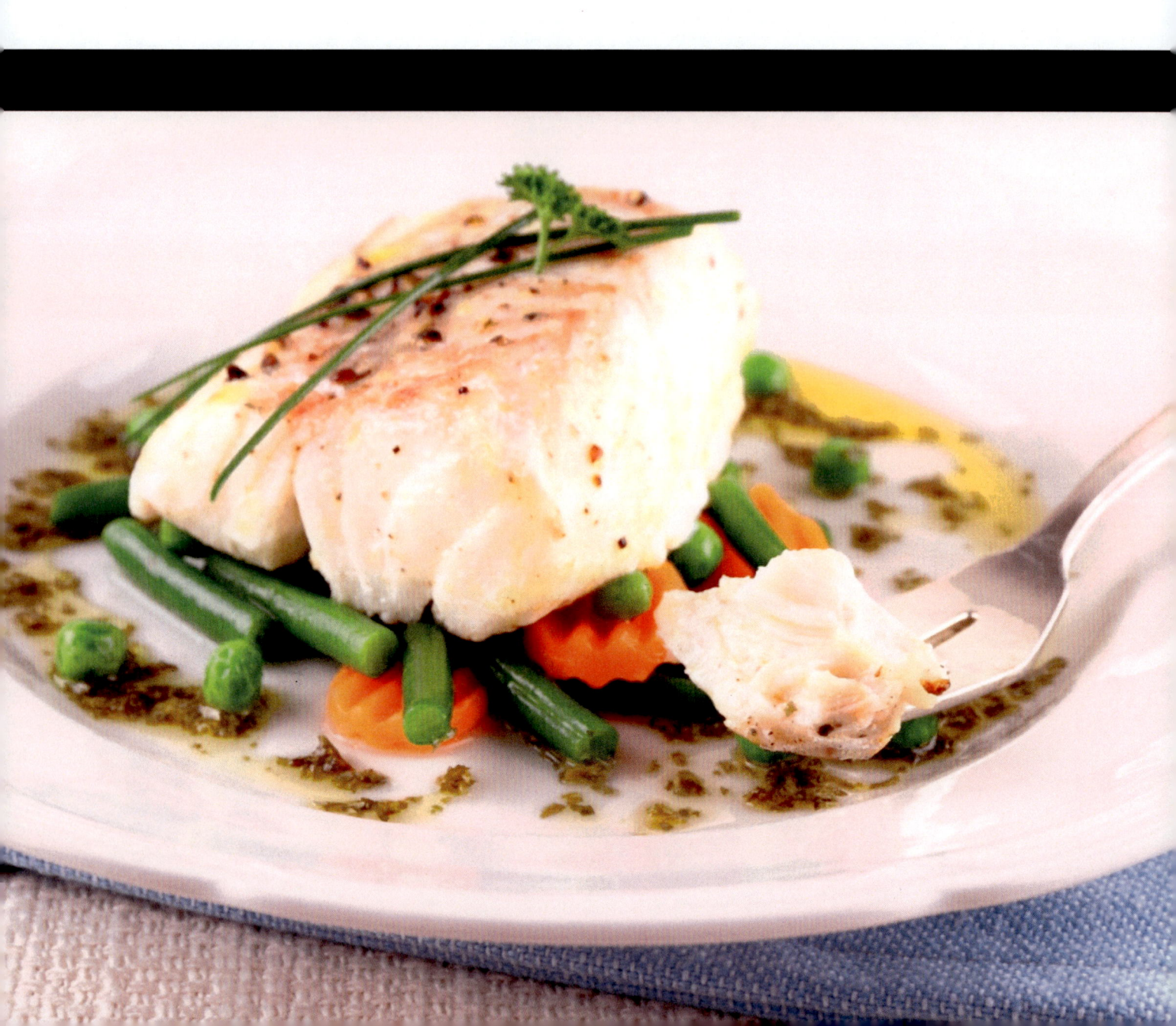

Directions

1. Preheat the oven's broiler and set the oven rack about 6 inches from the heat source. Line a broiler pan with aluminum foil.

2. Place the cod fillets on the foil, and brush with butter. Season with lemon juice, tarragon, and black pepper; sprinkle with sesame seeds.

3. Broil the fish in the preheated broiler until the flesh turns opaque and white, and the fish flakes easily, about 10 minutes.

SANE — Free Tools: SANESolution.com/Tools — Superfoods: store.SANESolution.com

Salmon

Salmon Cardamom

Total Time: 25 min
Prep: 15 min
Cook: 10 min

8 Servings
1 Nutrient-Dense Protein Per Serving
2 Whole-Food Fat Per Serving

Ingredients

- 2 teaspoons salt
- 1-1/4 teaspoons paprika
- 1-1/4 teaspoons ground cardamom
- 1-1/4 teaspoons ground coriander
- 3/4 teaspoon ground black pepper
- 1/3 cup extra virgin coconut oil
- 2 tablespoons and 2 teaspoons maple syrup
- 1-1/4 (2 pound) salmon fillet, cut into 3-inch pieces

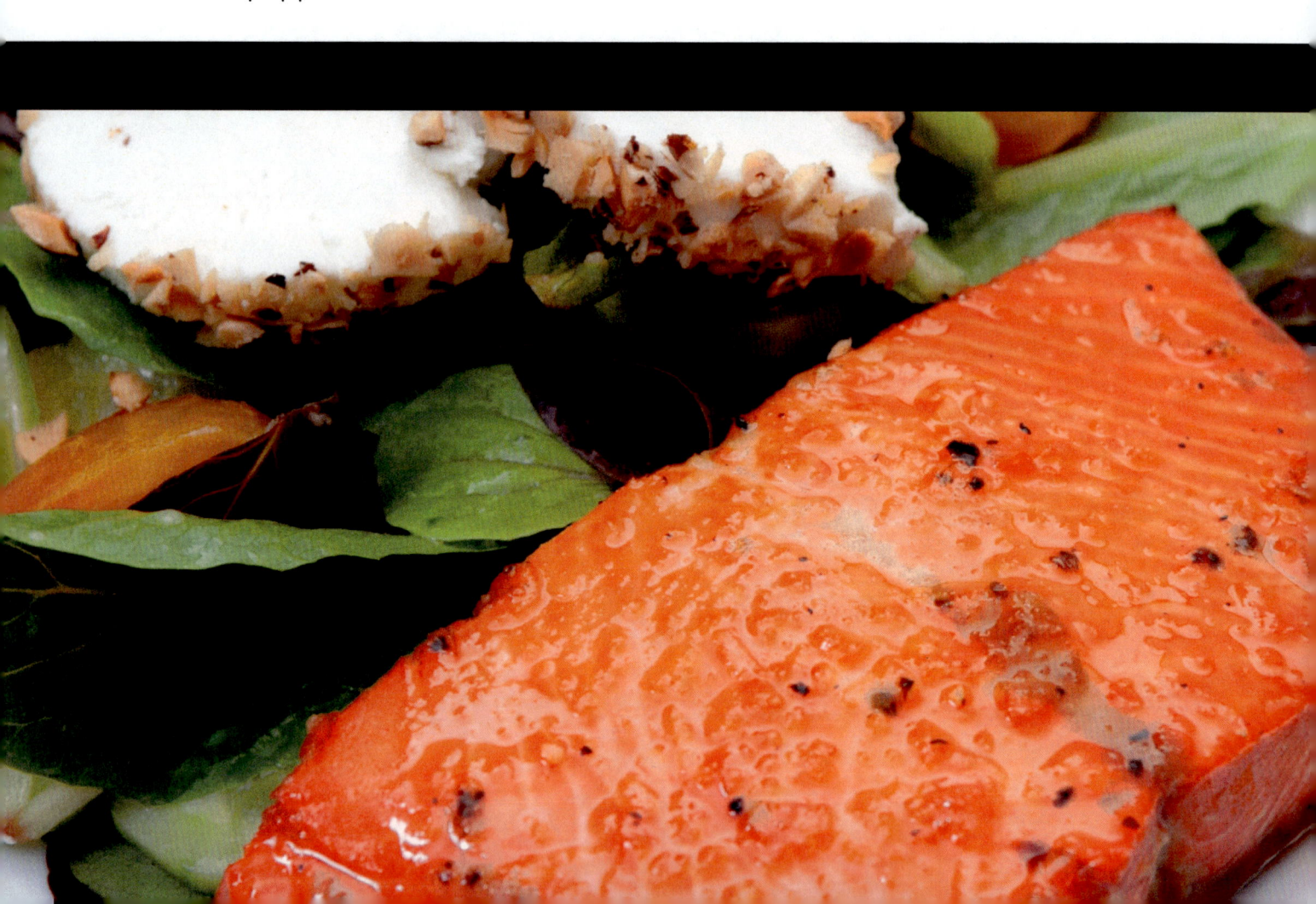

Directions

1. Stir salt, paprika, cardamom, coriander, and black pepper together in a bowl. Add melted oil and maple syrup and stir until evenly combined.

2. Preheat a non-stick frying pan over medium-high heat, about 350 degrees F (175 degrees C).

3. Dredge salmon pieces through the maple syrup mixture until evenly coated on all sides.

4. Cook salmon in the preheated pan until fish flakes easily with a fork, 5 to 7 minutes per side.

SANE   Free Tools: SANESolution.com/Tools   Superfoods: store.SANESolution.com

Hoisin Salmon

Total Time: 40 min
Prep: 10 min
Cook: 30 min

8 Servings
2 Nutrient-Dense Protein Per Serving
2 Whole-Food Fat Per Serving

Ingredients

- 1/4 cup and 3 tablespoons reduced-sodium soy sauce
- 1/3 cup hoisin sauce
- 1 tablespoon and 1 teaspoon chili garlic sauce
- 2 tablespoons and 2 teaspoons fresh lemon juice
- 1 tablespoon and 1 teaspoon grated fresh ginger root
- 1-1/4 cloves garlic, pressed
- 2 tablespoons and 2 teaspoons extra virgin coconut oil
- 8 (6 ounce) skinless, boneless salmon fillets

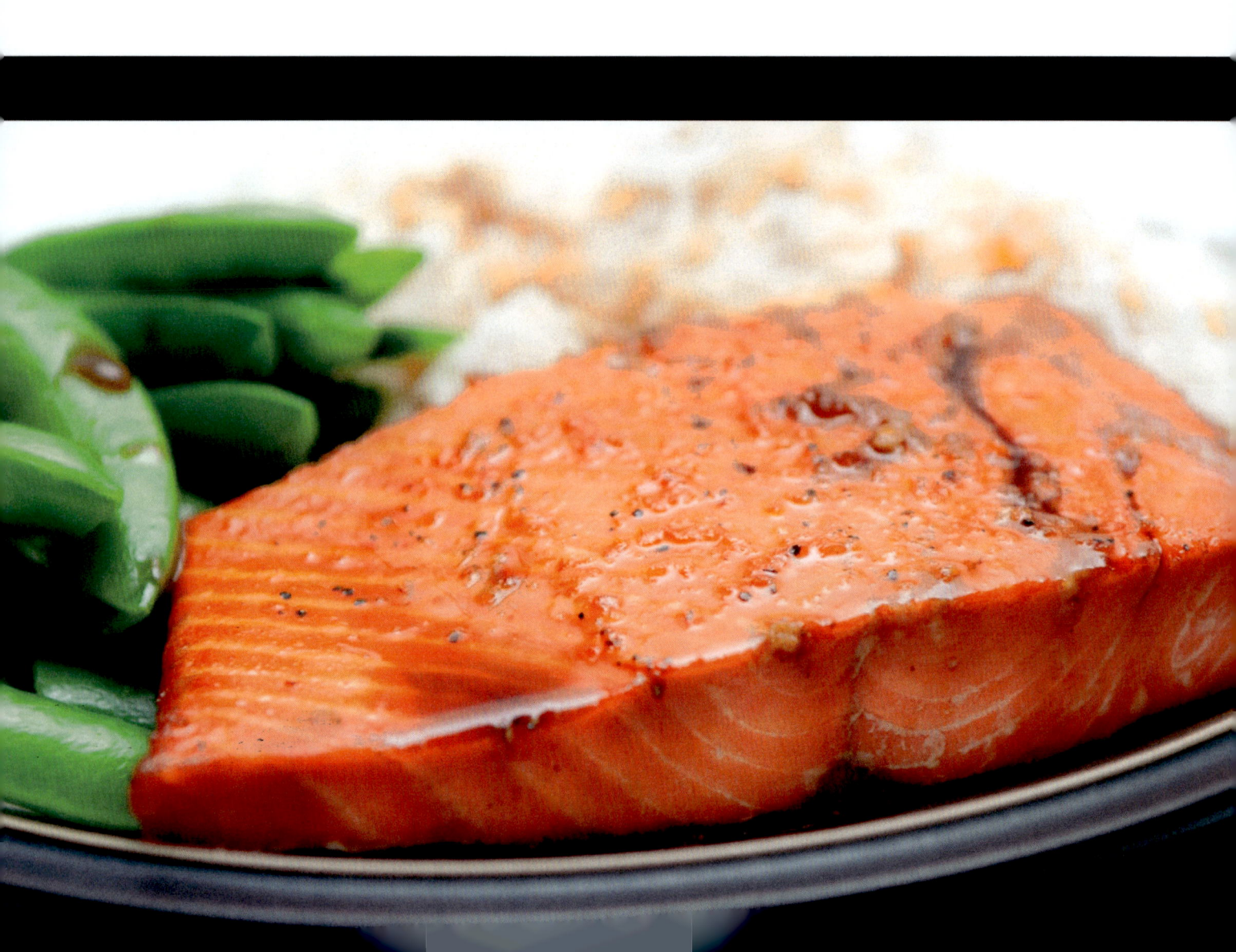

Directions

1. Whisk together the soy sauce, hoisin sauce, chili sauce, lemon juice, ginger, garlic, and extra virgin coconut oil in a 9×13 inch baking dish. Place the salmon fillets into the marinade, and turn to evenly coat. Cover the dish with plastic wrap, and marinate in the refrigerator for 30 minutes.

2. Preheat an oven to 350 degrees F (175 degrees C). Remove and discard the plastic wrap from the salmon, use a spoon to scoop up the marinade that has collected in the bottom of the baking dish, and drizzle it over the salmon fillets.

3. Bake in the preheated oven until the salmon flakes easily with a fork, about 30 minutes.

SANE Free Tools: SANESolution.com/Tools   Superfoods: store.SANESolution.com

Cilantro Salmon

Total Time: 30 min
Prep: 10 min
Cook: 20 min

8 Servings
2 Nutrient-Dense Protein Per Serving
2 Whole-Food Fat Per Serving

Ingredients

- 3 pounds salmon
- 1/4 cup butter
- 1 cup chopped cilantro
- 1 fresh jalapeno pepper, seeded and chopped
- Old Bay Seasoning TM to taste

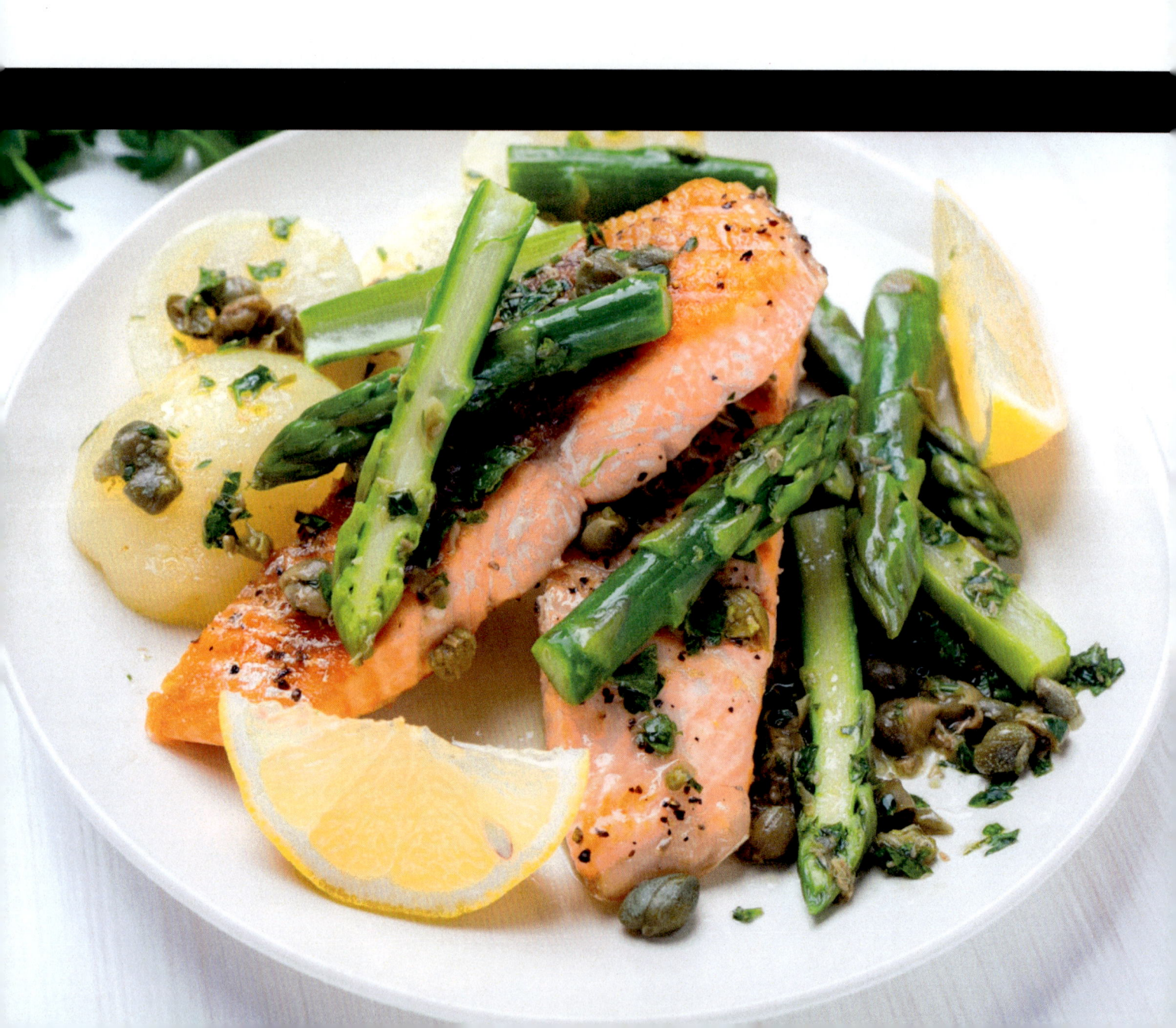

Directions

1. Preheat grill for high heat.

2. Lightly grease one side of a large sheet of aluminum foil. Place salmon on the greased side of foil. Melt the butter in a saucepan over medium heat. Remove from heat, and mix in cilantro and jalapeno. When cilantro is wilted, drizzle butter mixture over the salmon.

3. Place foil with salmon on the grill. Season with Old Bay. Cook 15 minutes, or until fish is easily flaked with a fork.

SANE Free Tools: SANESolution.com/Tools Superfoods: store.SANESolution.com

Moroccan Salmon

Total Time: 27 min
Prep: 15 min
Cook: 12 min

8 Servings
1 Nutrient-Dense Protein Per Serving
1 Whole-Food Fat Per Serving

Ingredients

- 1 teaspoon ground cinnamon
- 1 teaspoon ground cumin
- 3/4 teaspoon salt
- 3/4 teaspoon ground ginger
- 1/4 teaspoon mustard powder
- 1/4 teaspoon ground nutmeg
- 1/8 teaspoon cayenne pepper
- 1/8 teaspoon ground allspice
- 2-3/4 teaspoons white sugar
- 2-3/4 pounds (1-inch thick) boneless, skin-on center-cut salmon fillets
- 1 tablespoon and 1 teaspoon fresh lime juice

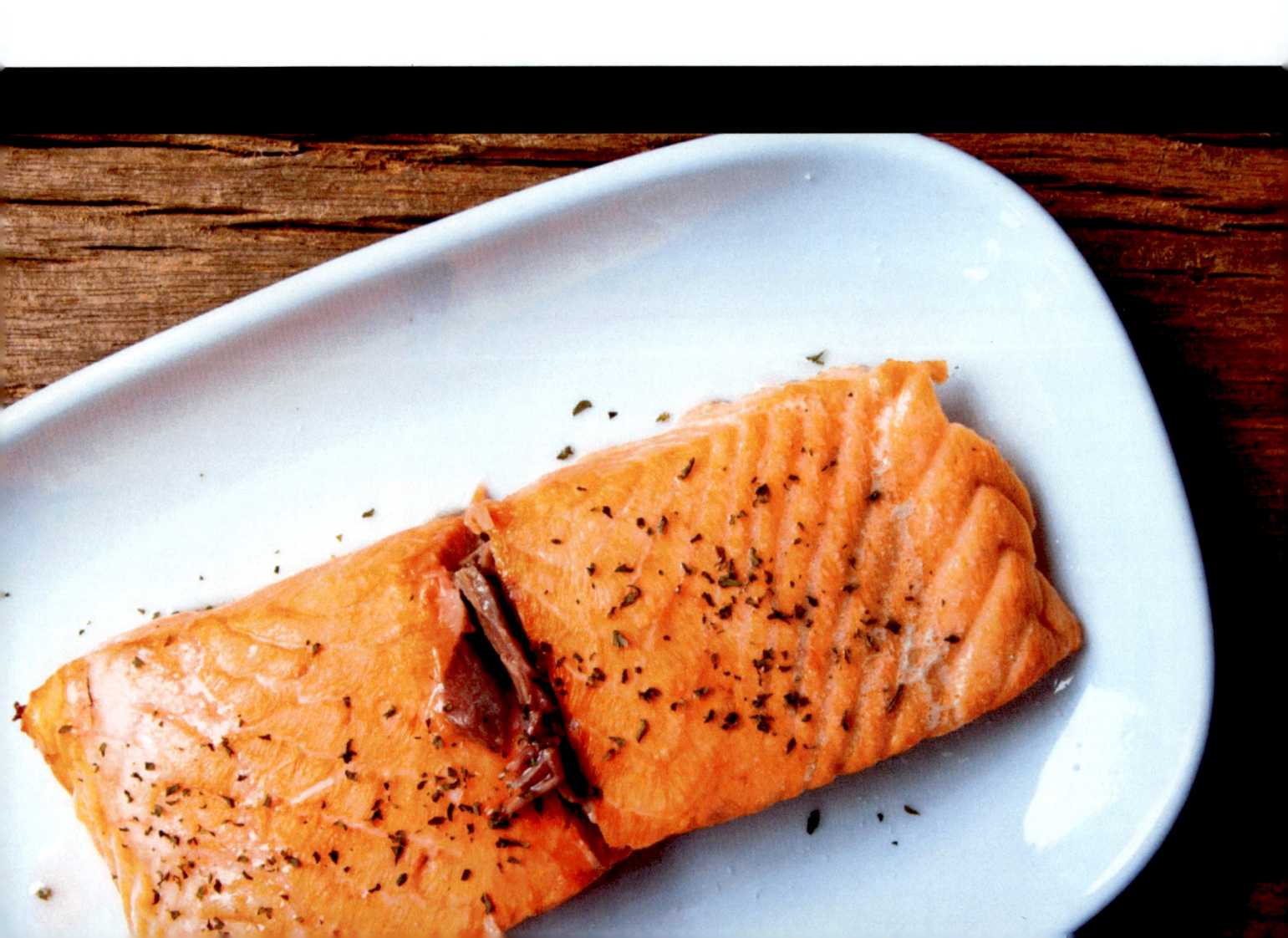

Directions

1. In a small bowl, combine the cinnamon, cumin, salt, ginger, mustard, nutmeg, cayenne, allspice, and sugar; set aside.

2. Line a baking sheet with foil, then spray with nonstick cooking spray. Rinse the salmon with cold water and pat dry. Lightly sprinkle the skin with the spice mix, then place the salmon skin-side down on the prepared baking sheet. Sprinkle the remaining spice mix evenly over the salmon. Allow the salmon to come to room temperature, 30 to 40 minutes.

3. Preheat oven to 425 degrees F (220 degrees C).

4. Sprinkle the salmon with lime juice and roast in the oven for 12 minutes. Remove from oven and allow to stand at room temperature for 15 minutes. The salmon will still be rare when removed from the oven, but will continue to cook as it rests. After 15 minutes, wrap the fish tightly with foil and refrigerate for at least 2 hours before serving.

SANE Free Tools: SANESolution.com/Tools   Superfoods: store.SANESolution.com

Scrumptious Baked Salmon

Total Time: 40 min
Prep: 15 min
Cook: 25 min

8 Servings
1 Nutrient-Dense Protein Per Serving
1 Whole-Food Fat Per Serving

Ingredients

- 4 (8 ounce) salmon fillets
- salt and ground black pepper to taste
- 1 cup chopped basil leaves
- extra virgin coconut oil cooking spray
- 4 lemon, thinly sliced

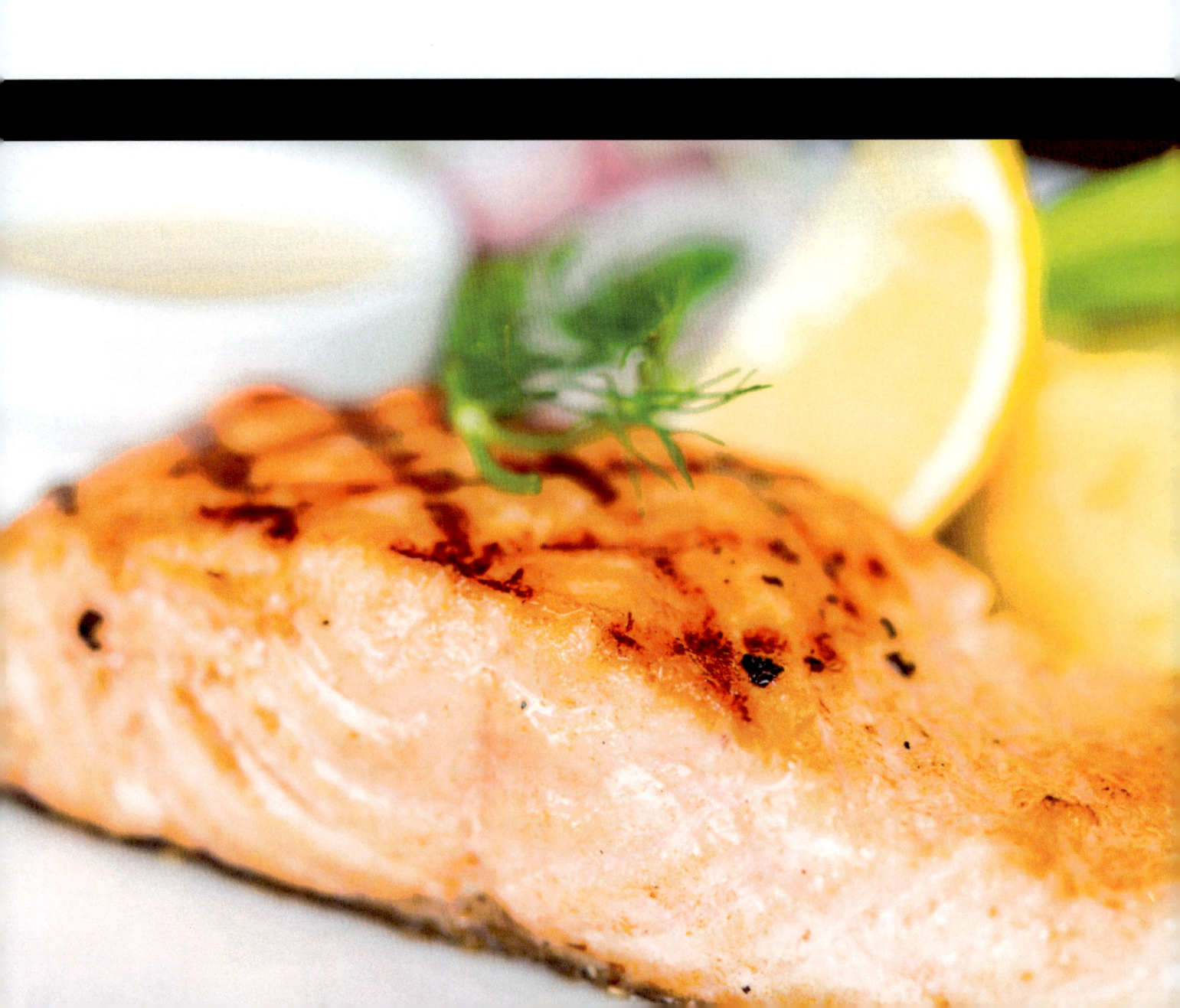

Directions

1. Place an oven rack in the lowest position in oven and preheat oven to 400 degrees F (200 degrees C).

2. Place salmon fillet with skin side down in the middle of a large piece of parchment paper; season with salt and black pepper. Cut 2 3-inch slits into the fish with a sharp knife. Stuff chopped basil leaves into the slits. Spray fillet with cooking spray and arrange lemon slices on top.

3. Fold edges of parchment paper over the fish several times to seal into an airtight packet. Place sealed packet onto a baking sheet.

4. Bake fish on the bottom rack of oven until salmon flakes easily and meat is pink and opaque with an interior of slightly darker pink color, about 25 minutes. An instant-read meat thermometer inserted into the thickest part of the fillet should read at least 145 degrees F (65 degrees C). To serve, cut the parchment paper open and remove lemon slices before plating fish.

Salmon Bake

Total Time: 35 min
Prep: 15 min
Cook: 20 min

8 Servings
1 Non Starchy Vegetables Per Serving
2 Nutrient-Dense Protein Per Serving
1 Whole-Food Fat Per Serving

Ingredients

- 4 pounds salmon fillet, halved
- 4 small tomato, chopped
- 20 green onions, chopped
- 1 teaspoon salt
- 1 teaspoon pepper

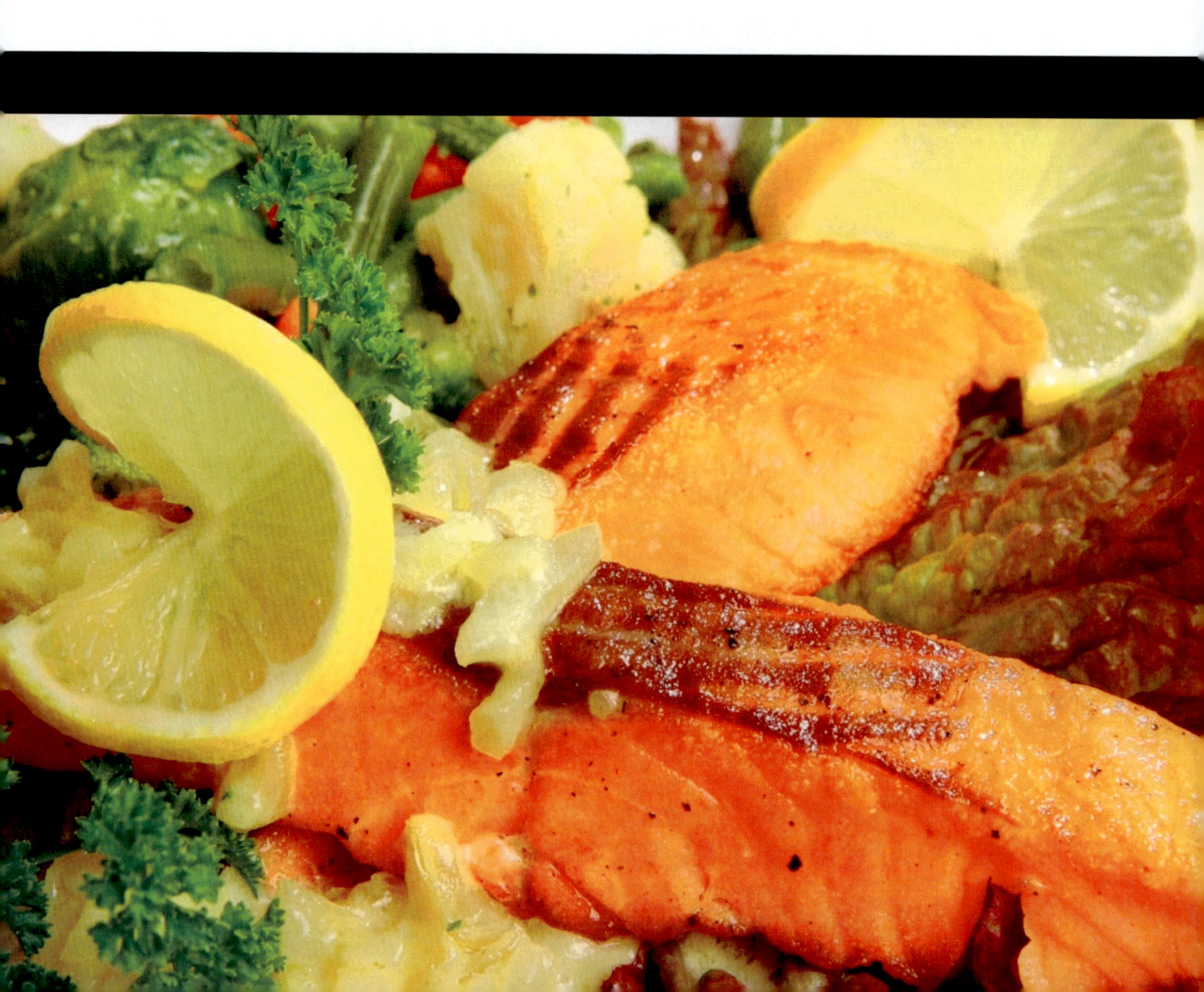

Directions

1. Preheat oven to 350 degrees F (175 degrees C).

2. Place salmon on a lightly oiled sheet pan or in a shallow baking dish, folding under thin outer edges of fillets for even cooking. Top salmon with chopped tomatoes and green onions, and season with salt and pepper.

3. Cook salmon in the preheated oven, uncovered, for approximately 20 minutes. Fish is done when easily flaked with a fork.

Orange-Ginger Salmon

Total Time: 50 min
Prep: 20 min
Cook: 30 min

8 Servings
2 Nutrient-Dense Protein Per Serving
1 Whole-Food Fat Per Serving

Ingredients

- 3-1/4 pounds salmon fillet
- 1-1/2 cups and 2 tablespoons orange juice
- 1 tablespoon and 1/4 teaspoon balsamic vinegar
- 1-1/2 teaspoons finely chopped fresh ginger root
- salt and ground black pepper to taste

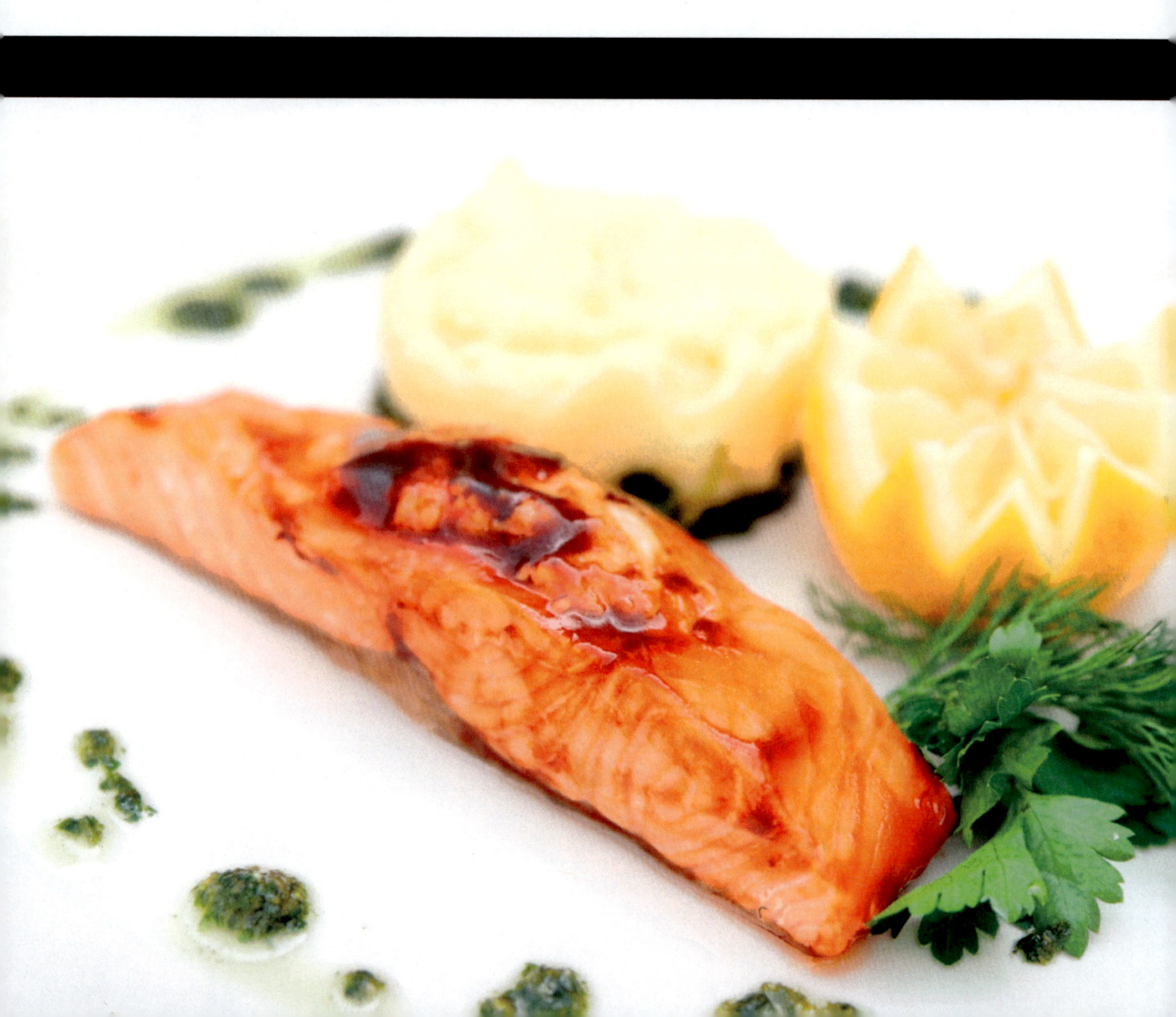

Directions

1. Preheat oven to 400 degrees F (200 degrees C).

2. Place orange juice in a small saucepan over medium low heat. Cook and stir 10 to 15 minutes, until reduced by about 1/2 and thickened. Remove from heat, and allow to cool.

3. Stir balsamic vinegar and ginger root into orange juice.

4. Line a medium baking dish with parchment paper. Place salmon fillet on paper, skin side down. Season with salt and pepper. Cover with 1/2 the orange juice mixture.

5. Bake salmon in the preheated oven 10 to 15 minutes. Brush with remaining marinade, and continue baking 10 to 15 minutes, until easily flaked with a fork.

SANE   Free Tools: SANESolution.com/Tools   Superfoods: store.SANESolution.com

Pan Seared Salmon

Total Time: 20 min
Prep: 10 min
Cook: 10 min

8 Servings
2 Nutrient-Dense Protein Per Serving
2 Whole-Food Fat Per Serving

Ingredients

- 8 (6 ounce) fillets salmon
- 1/4 cup extra virgin coconut oil
- 1/4 cup capers
- 1/4 teaspoon salt
- 1/4 teaspoon ground black pepper
- 8 slices lemon

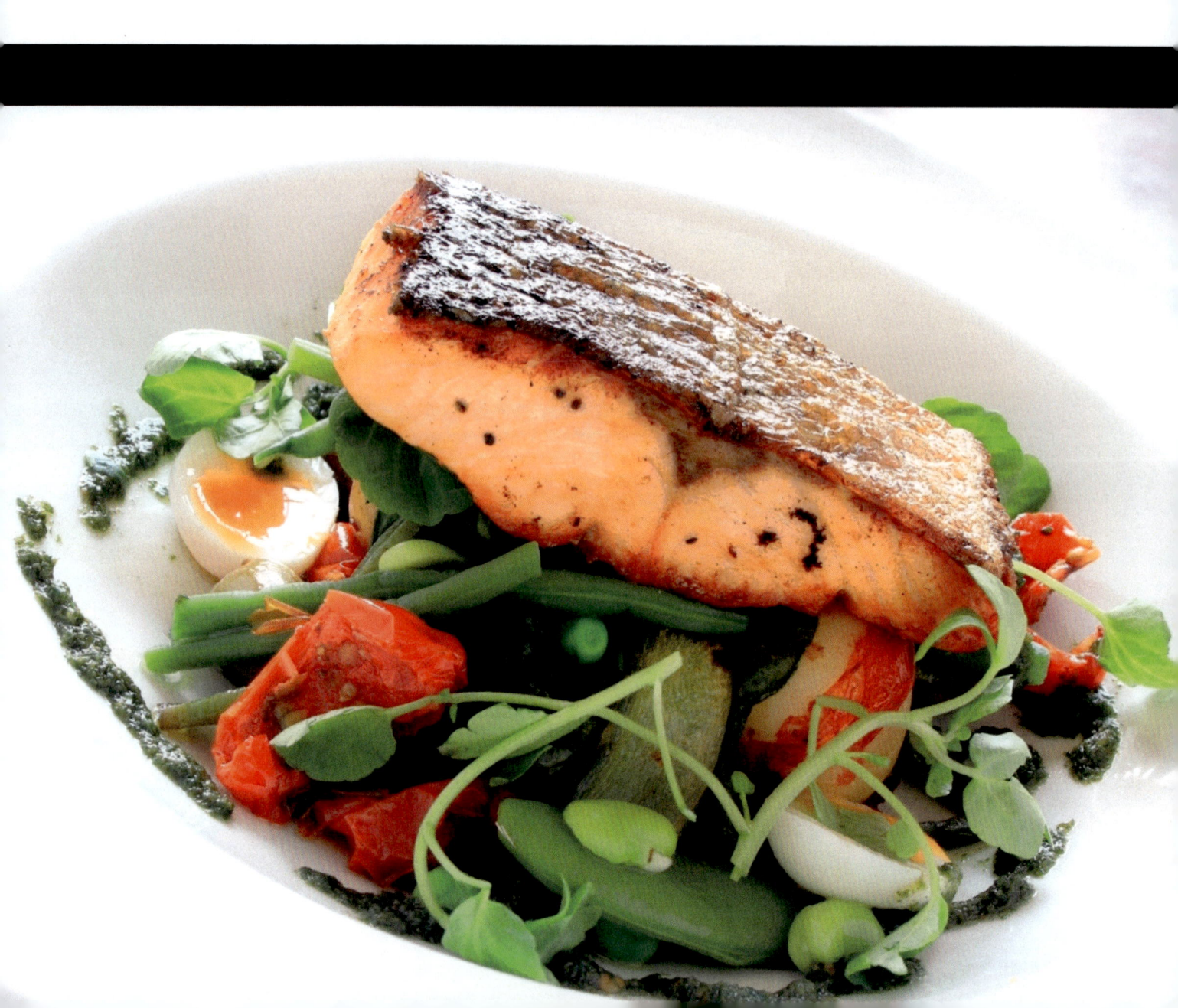

Directions

1. Preheat a large heavy skillet over medium heat for 3 minutes.

2. Coat salmon with melted extra virgin coconut oil. Place in skillet, and increase heat to high. Cook for 3 minutes. Sprinkle with capers, and salt and pepper. Turn salmon over, and cook for 5 minutes, or until browned. Salmon is done when it flakes easily with a fork.

3. Transfer salmon to individual plates, and garnish with lemon slices.

Garlic Salmon

Total Time: 40 min
Prep: 15 min
Cook: 25 min

8 Servings
1 Nutrient-Dense Protein Per Serving
1 Whole-Food Fat Per Serving

Ingredients

- 2 pounds salmon fillet
- salt and pepper to taste
- 4 cloves garlic, minced
- 1-1/4 sprigs fresh dill, chopped
- 6-3/4 slices lemon
- 6-3/4 sprigs fresh dill weed
- 2-3/4 green onions, chopped

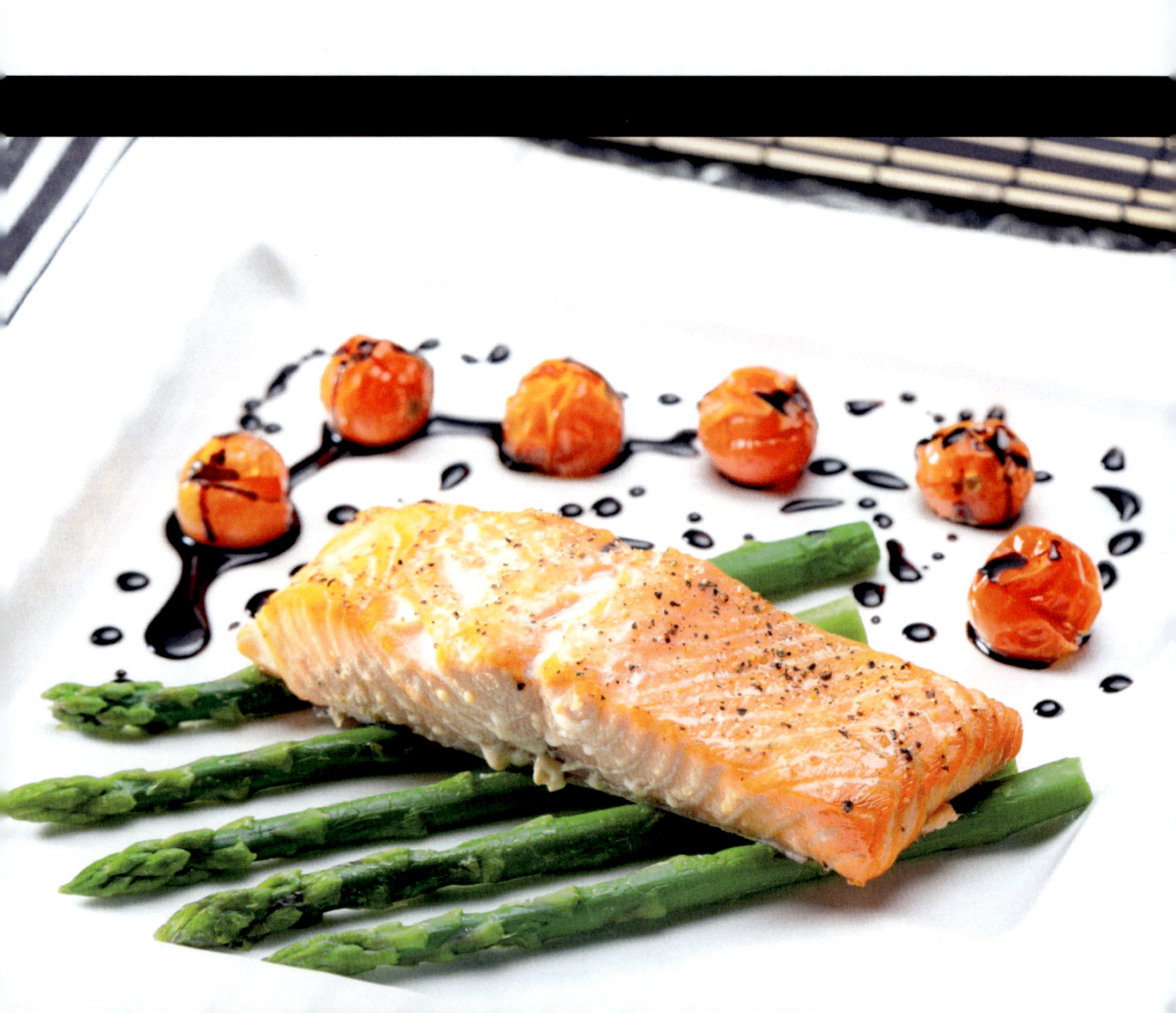

Directions

1. Preheat oven to 450 degrees F (230 degrees C). Spray two large pieces of aluminum foil with cooking spray.

2. Place salmon fillet on top of one piece of foil. Sprinkle salmon with salt, pepper, garlic and chopped dill. Arrange lemon slices on top of fillet and place a sprig of dill on top of each lemon slice. Sprinkle fillet with chopped scallions.

3. Cover salmon with second piece of foil and pinch together foil to tightly seal. Place on a baking sheet or in a large baking dish.

4. Bake in preheated oven for 20 to 25 minutes, until salmon flakes easily.

SANE — Free Tools: SANESolution.com/Tools — Superfoods: store.SANESolution.com

Garlic and Dill Salmon

Total Time: 35 min
Prep: 10 min
Cook: 25 min

8 Servings
1 Nutrient-Dense Protein Per Serving
2 Whole-Food Fat Per Serving

Ingredients

- 2 pounds salmon fillets
- 1/2 cup butter, melted
- 1/2 cup and 2 tablespoons lemon juice
- 2 tablespoons dried dill weed
- 1/2 teaspoon garlic powder
- sea salt to taste
- freshly ground black pepper to taste

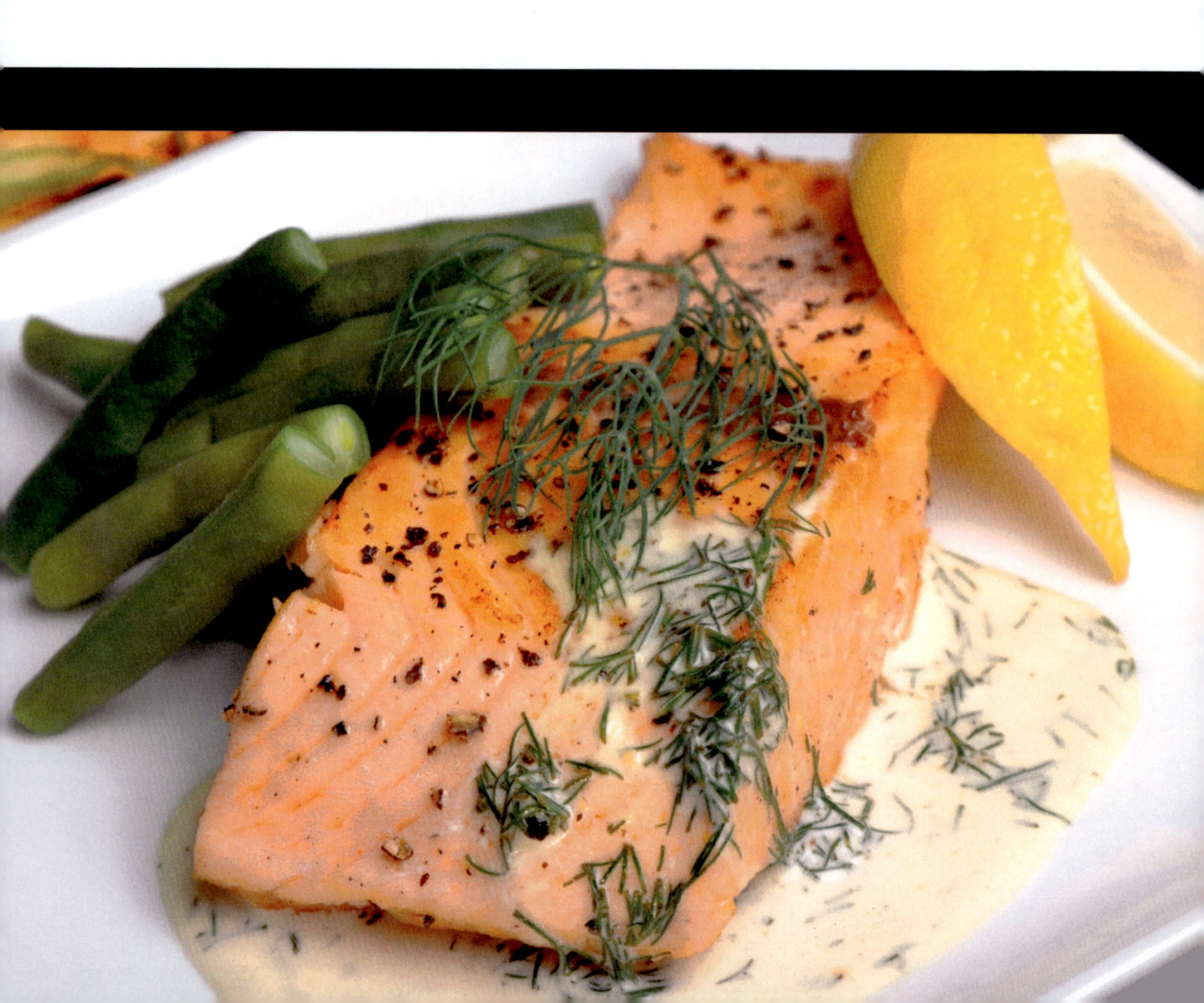

Directions

1. Preheat oven to 350 degrees F (175 degrees C). Lightly grease a medium baking dish.

2. Place salmon in the baking dish. Mix the butter and lemon juice in a small bowl, and drizzle over the salmon. Season with dill, garlic powder, sea salt, and pepper.

3. Bake 25 minutes in the preheated oven, or until salmon is easily flaked with a fork.

SANE   Free Tools: SANESolution.com/Tools   Superfoods: store.SANESolution.com

Spiced Garlic Salmon

Total Time: 25 min
Prep: 10 min
Cook: 15 min

8 Servings
1 Nutrient-Dense Protein Per Serving
2 Whole-Food Fat Per Serving

Ingredients

- 8 cloves garlic, crushed
- 4 dried red chile pepper
- 1/4 cup extra virgin coconut oil
- 1 tablespoon and 1 teaspoon whole grain mustard
- 1/2 cup fresh lime juice
- sea salt to taste
- freshly ground black pepper
- 8 (6 ounce) fillets salmon

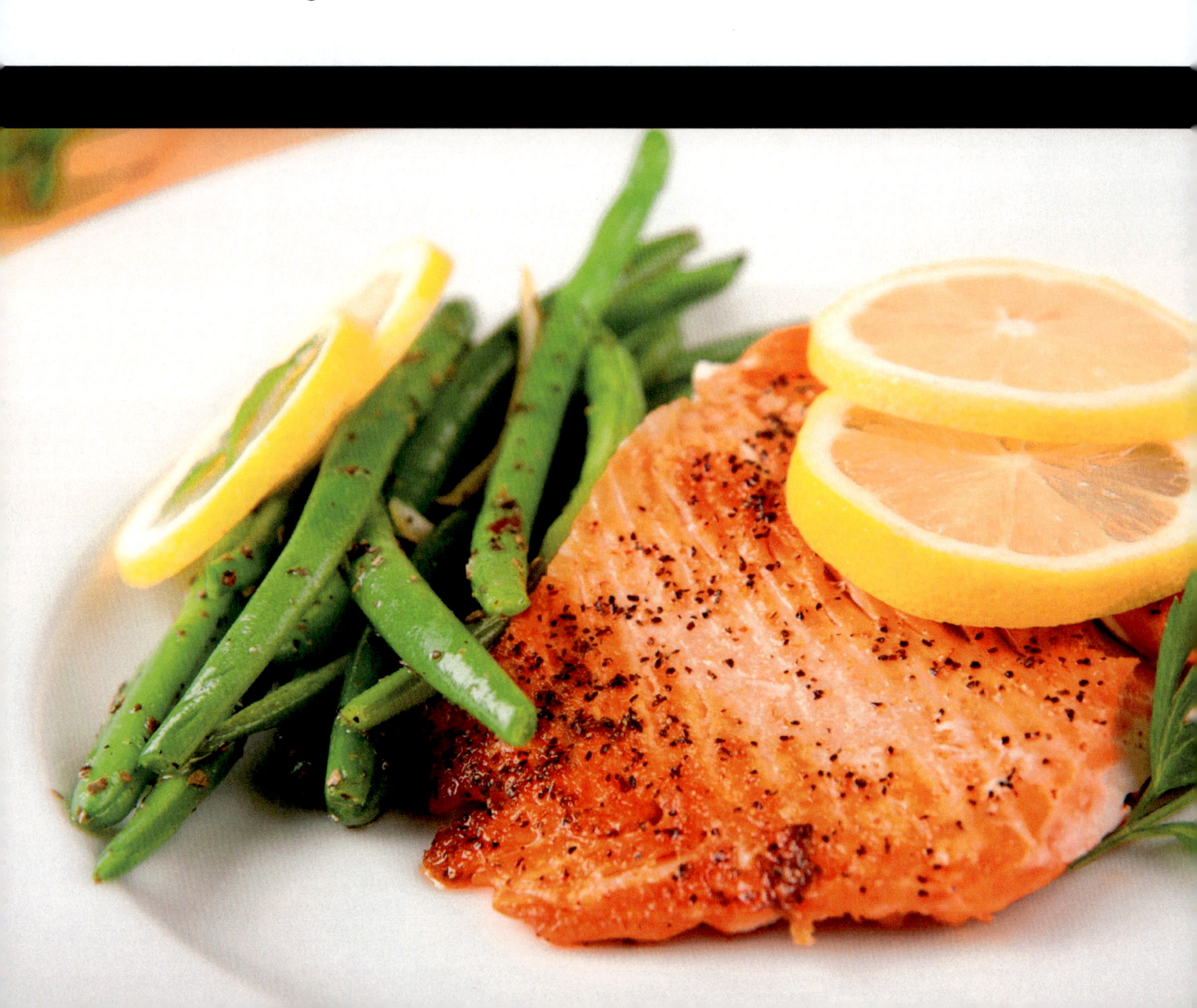

Directions

1. Preheat oven to 400 degrees F (200 degrees C). Line a medium baking dish with aluminum foil. Lightly grease foil.

2. Grind together the garlic, chile pepper, and melted extra virgin coconut oil. Mix into a thick paste with the mustard, lime juice, salt, and pepper. Place the salmon fillets in the prepared baking dish, and coat with the paste mixture.

3. Bake salmon 12 to 15 minutes in the preheated oven, or until fish is easily flaked with a fork.

Roast Balsamic Salmon

Total Time: 25 min
Prep: 10 min
Cook: 15 min

8 Servings
1 Nutrient-Dense Protein Per Serving
2 Whole-Food Fat Per Serving

Ingredients

- 1/4 cup packed brown sugar
- 1/4 cup balsamic vinegar
- 2 tablespoons extra virgin coconut oil
- 1/2 teaspoon dried rosemary
- 2 cloves garlic, minced
- 1/2 teaspoon ground black pepper
- 3 pounds salmon fillets
- 1 teaspoon salt

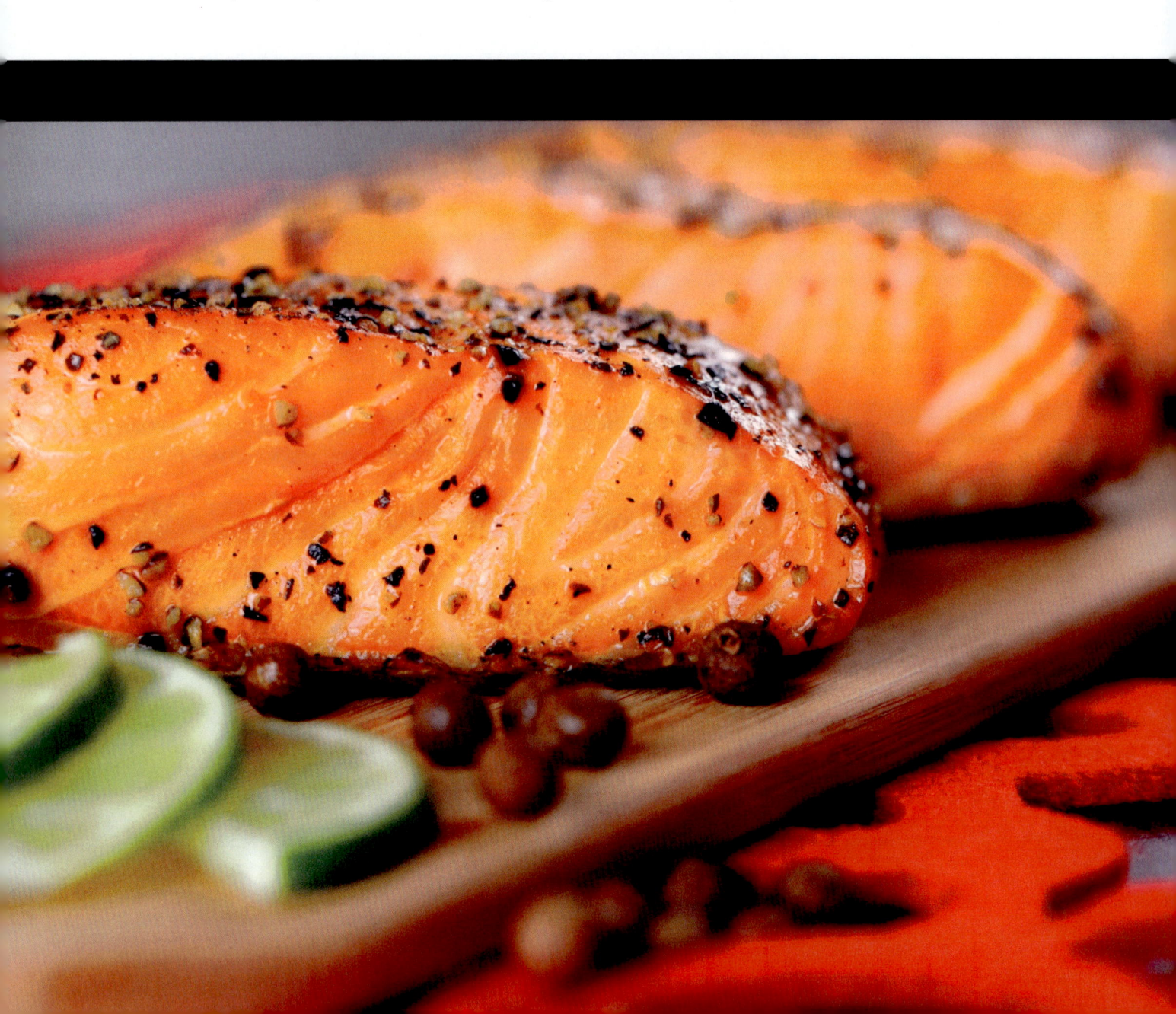

Directions

1. Whisk together the brown sugar, balsamic vinegar, extra virgin coconut oil, rosemary, garlic, and pepper in a large bowl. Reserve 1 tablespoon of marinade in a small bowl, and set aside. Add the salmon and toss to evenly coat. Cover the bowl with plastic wrap, and marinate in the refrigerator for 30 minutes. Remove the salmon from the marinade, and shake off excess. Place salmon in an aluminum foil-lined baking dish, and sprinkle with salt.

2. Preheat an oven to 450 degrees F (230 degrees C).

3. Roast in the preheated oven until the fish is easily flaked with a fork, about 10 minutes. Brush salmon with the reserved marinade, and return to the oven. Roast until glazed, about 1 minute.

S∆NE   Free Tools: SANESolution.com/Tools   Superfoods: store.SANESolution.com

Cedar Salmon

Total Time: 35 min
Prep: 15 min
Cook: 20 min

8 Servings
1 Nutrient-Dense Protein Per Serving
3 Whole-Food Fat Per Serving

Ingredients

- 1 (3 pound) whole filet of salmon, skin on, scored (up to but not through the skin) into serving pieces
- 6 tablespoons extra virgin coconut oil
- 4 large garlic cloves, minced
- 1/4 cup minced fresh dill
- 2 teaspoons salt
- 1 teaspoon ground black pepper
- 1 teaspoon lemon zest, plus lemon wedges for serving

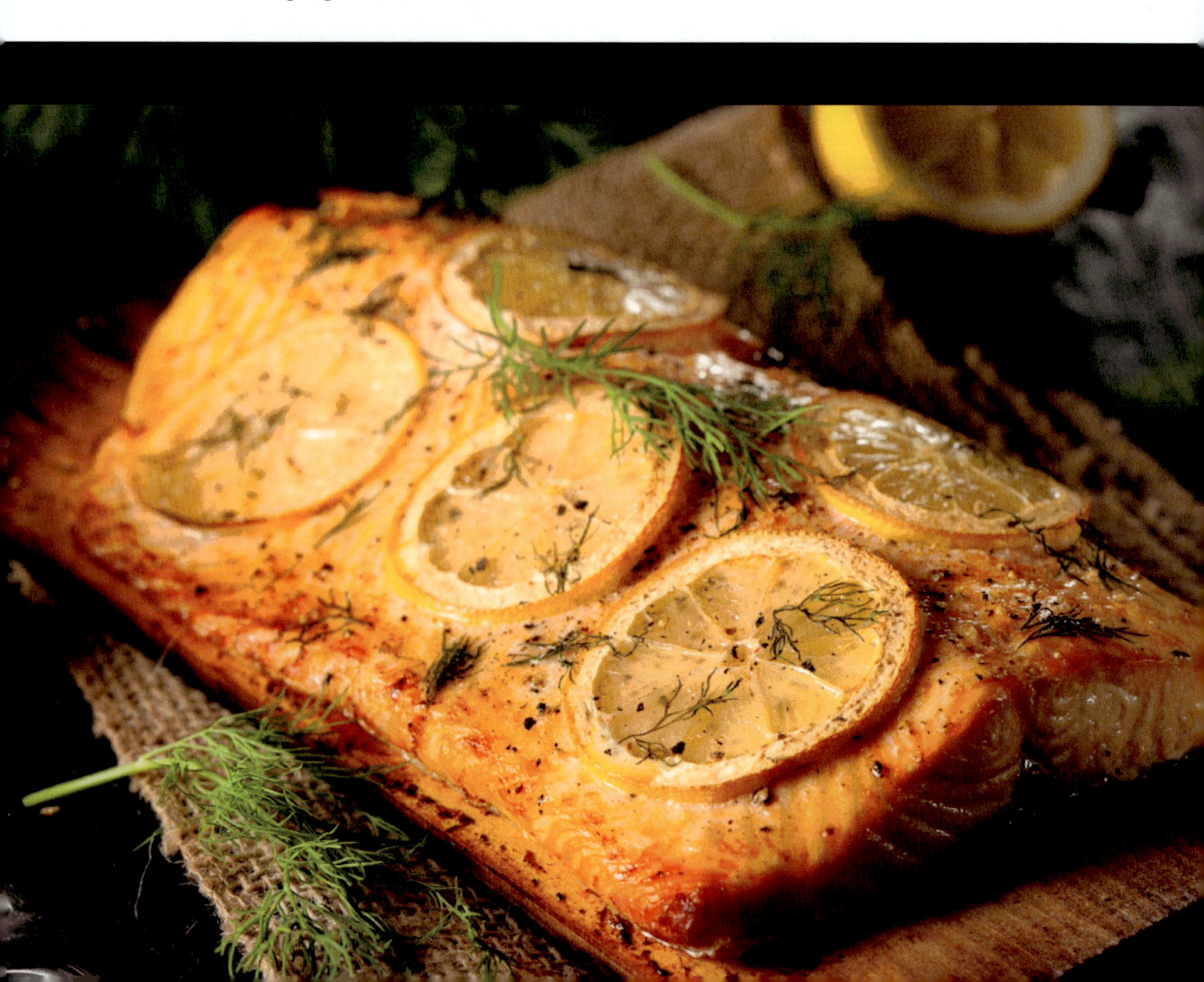

Directions

1. Soak an untreated cedar plank (or planks) large enough to hold a side of salmon (5 to 7 inches wide and 16 to 20 inches long) in water, weighting it with something heavy, like a brick, so it stays submerged 30 minutes to 24 hours.

2. When ready to grill, either build a charcoal fire in half the grill or turn grill burners on high for 10 minutes. Meanwhile, mix melted oil, garlic, dill, salt, pepper and lemon zest; rub over salmon and into scored areas to coat.

3. Place soaked cedar on hot grill grate, close lid, and watch until wood starts to smoke, about 5 minutes. Transfer salmon to hot plank, move salmon off direct charcoal heat or turn burners to low, and cook covered until salmon is just opaque throughout (130 on a meat thermometer inserted in the thickest section) 20 to 25 minutes or longer, depending on thickness and grill temperature. Let sit 5 minutes; serve with lemon wedges.

SANE Free Tools: SANESolution.com/Tools   Superfoods: store.SANESolution.com

Balsamic Salmon

Total Time: 40 min
Prep: 10 min
Cook: 30 min

8 Servings
1 Nutrient-Dense Protein Per Serving
2 Whole-Food Fat Per Serving

Ingredients

- 8 (4 ounce) skinless, boneless salmon fillets
- 1 cup vegan margarine (such as Smart Balance®), melted
- 2 lemon, halved
- 1/2 cup balsamic vinegar
- 1/4 cup soy sauce
- 1/4 cup white sugar
- 1 teaspoon minced garlic
- 1 cup chopped fresh parsley

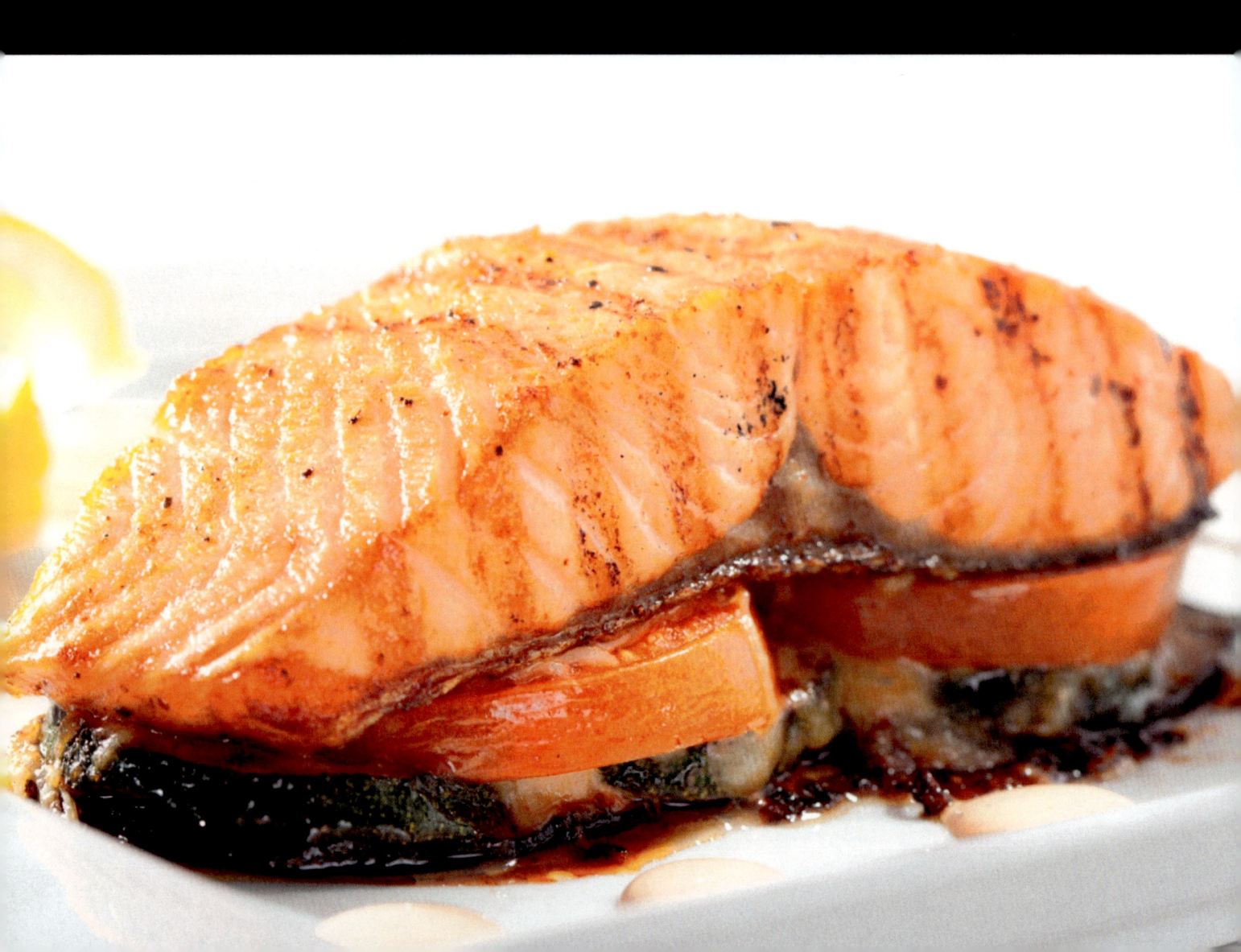

Directions

1. Preheat oven to 375 degrees F (190 degrees C).

2. Dip salmon fillets in melted margarine, covering both sides. Place in a baking dish. Squeeze lemons evenly over each fillet.

3. Whisk balsamic vinegar, soy sauce, sugar, and garlic together in a bowl; spoon over salmon fillets. Sprinkle with parsley; drizzle any remaining butter over fillets.

4. Bake in the preheated oven until fish is opaque and flakes easily with a fork, about 30 minutes. Remove from oven and cover with aluminum foil for 3 minutes before serving.

Garlic Balsamic Salmon

Total Time: 30 min
Prep: 10 min
Cook: 20 min

8 Servings
1 Nutrient-Dense Protein Per Serving
2 Whole-Food Fat Per Serving

Ingredients

- 8 (5 ounce) salmon fillets
- 5-1/4 cloves garlic, minced
- 1 tablespoon and 1 teaspoon white wine
- 1 tablespoon and 1 teaspoon honey
- 1/4 cup and 3 tablespoons balsamic vinegar
- 1 tablespoon and 2-1/4 teaspoons Dijon mustard
- salt and pepper to taste
- 1 tablespoon and 1 teaspoon chopped fresh oregano

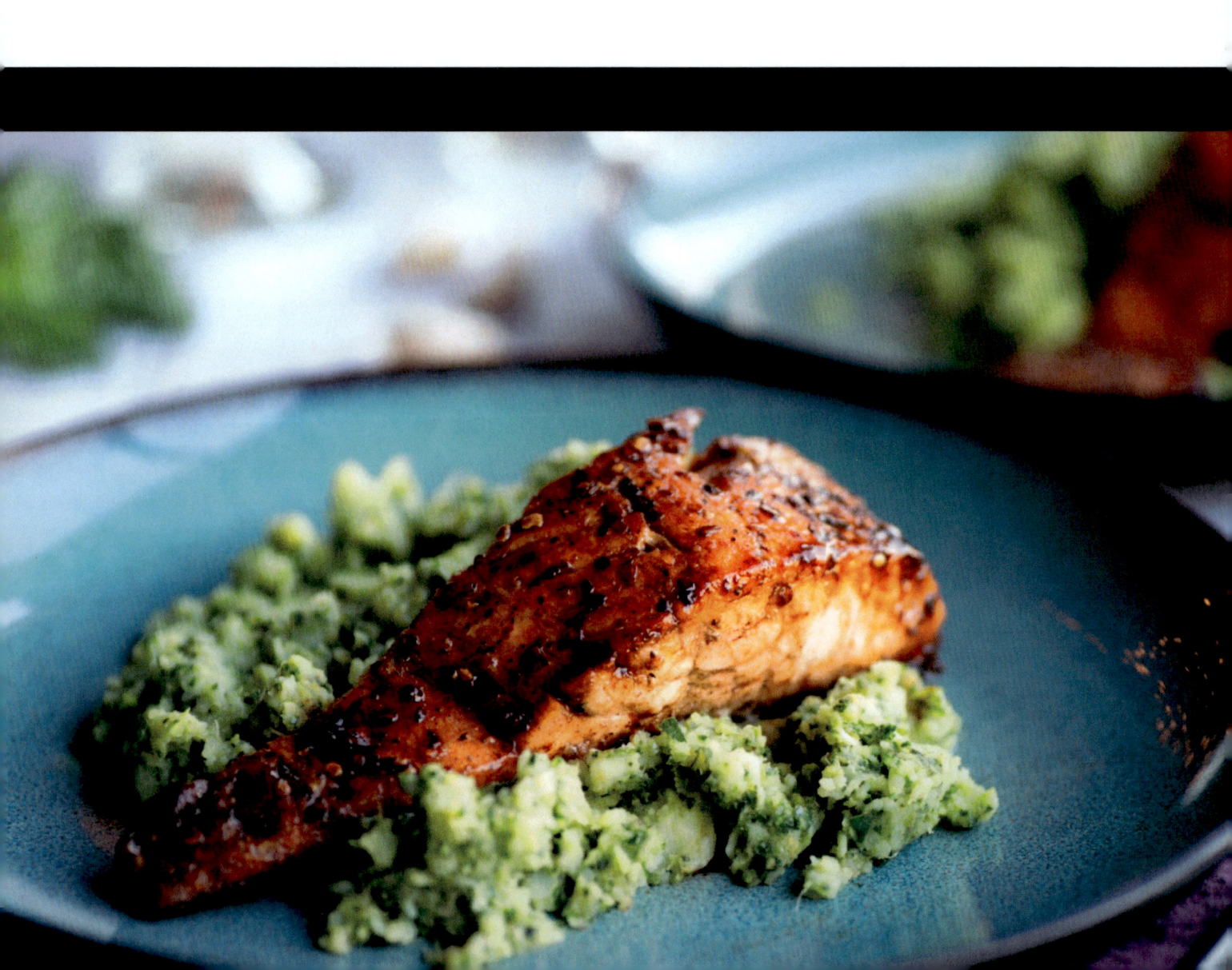

Directions

1. Preheat oven to 400 degrees F (200 degrees C). Line a baking sheet with aluminum foil, and spray with non-stick cooking spray.

2. Coat a small saucepan with non-stick cooking spray. Over medium heat, cook and stir garlic until soft, about 3 minutes. Mix in white wine, honey, balsamic vinegar, mustard, and salt and pepper. Simmer, uncovered, for about 3 minutes, or until slightly thickened.

3. Arrange salmon fillets on foil-lined baking sheet. Brush fillets with balsamic glaze, and sprinkle with oregano.

4. Bake in preheated oven for 10 to 14 minutes, or until flesh flakes easily with a fork. Brush fillets with remaining glaze, and season with salt and pepper. Use a spatula to transfer fillets to serving platter, leaving the skin behind on the foil.

SANE Free Tools: SANESolution.com/Tools   Superfoods: store.SANESolution.com

17 Minute Succulent Salmon

Total Time: 17 min
Prep: 7 min
Cook: 10 min

8 Servings
1 Nutrient-Dense Protein Per Serving
2 Whole-Food Fat Per Serving

Ingredients

- 1/2 cup butter
- 1/2 cup white wine
- 2 tablespoons lemon juice
- 2 tablespoons dried dill weed
- 2 teaspoons white sugar
- salt and ground black pepper to taste
- 8 salmon fillets

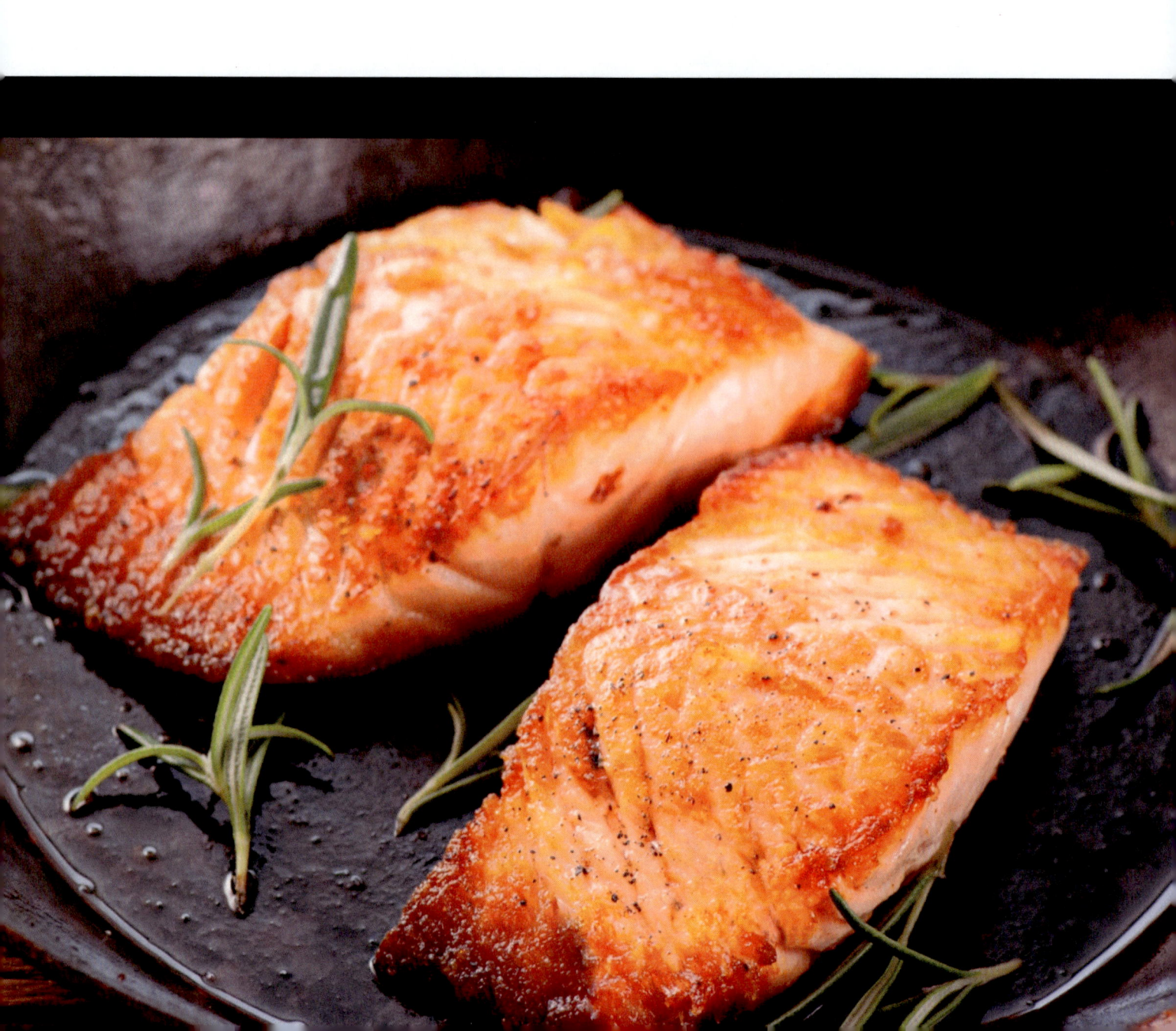

Directions

1. Combine butter, wine, lemon juice, dill, sugar, salt, and black pepper together in a microwave-safe casserole dish; place cover on dish.

2. Microwave butter mixture until butter is melted, 45 to 60 seconds. Add salmon, skin-side up, to butter mixture and place cover on dish. Microwave until salmon flakes easily with a fork, about 6 minutes.

SANE   Free Tools: SANESolution.com/Tools   Superfoods: store.SANESolution.com

India Salmon

Total Time: 30 min
Prep: 15 min
Cook: 15 min

8 Servings
2 Nutrient-Dense Protein Per Serving
2 Whole-Food Fat Per Serving

Ingredients

- 2 cups fat-free plain yogurt
- 1 tablespoon cayenne pepper
- 12 cloves garlic, minced
- 4 (2 inch) pieces fresh ginger root, minced
- 1/4 cup cilantro, finely chopped
- 2 tablespoons ground coriander seed
- 2 teaspoons ground cumin
- 2 teaspoons salt
- 1/2 teaspoon ground turmeric
- 8 (6 ounce) skinless, boneless salmon fillets

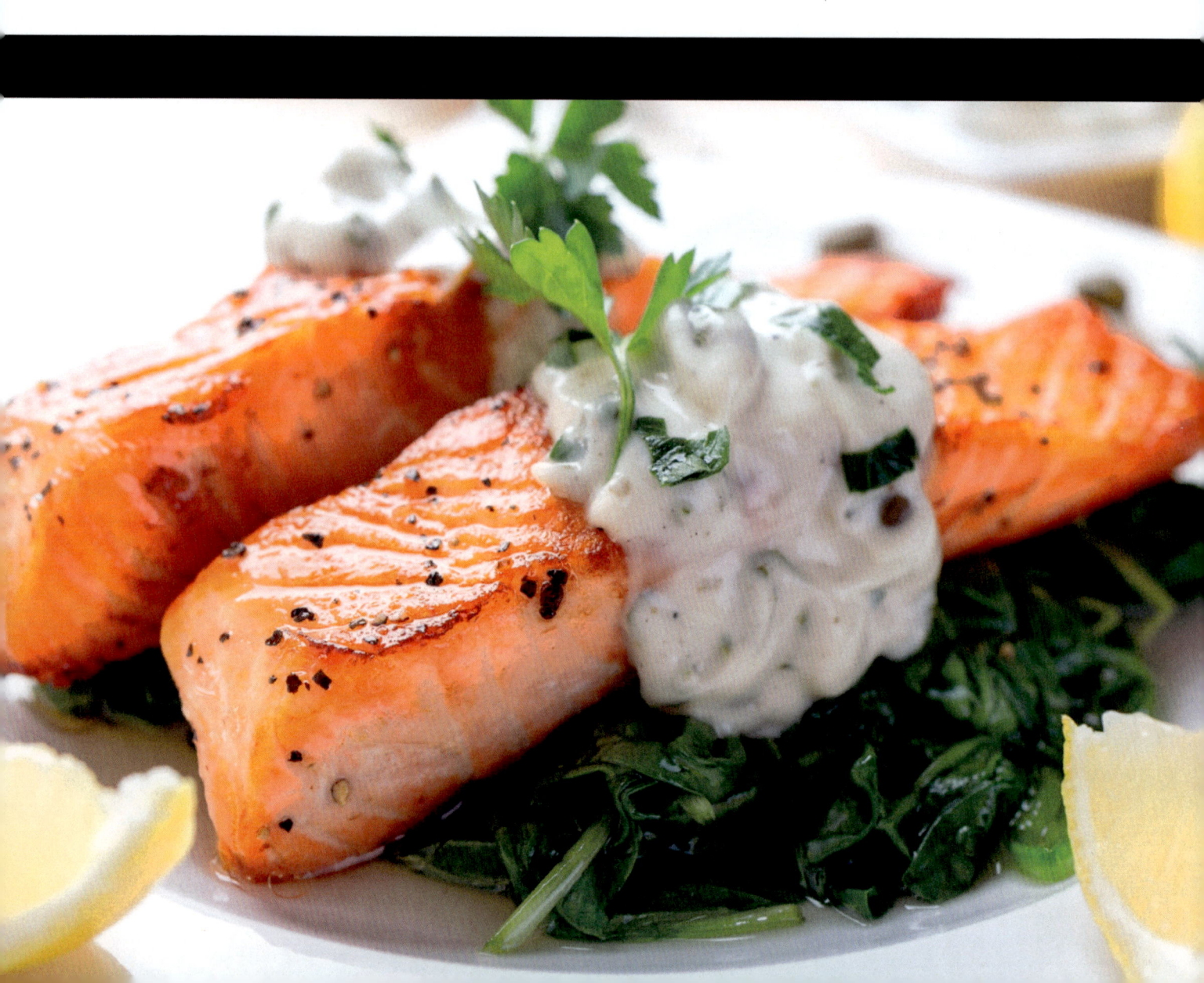

Directions

1. Combine the yogurt, cayenne pepper, garlic, ginger, cilantro, ground coriander, cumin, salt and turmeric in a resealable plastic bag. Close bag and mix everything together until evenly combined. Add the salmon and toss until well coated with the marinade; marinate overnight.

2. Preheat the oven broiler. Lightly grease a baking pan.

3. Remove salmon from marinade and shake off excess; discard remaining marinade. Place onto prepared baking pan and broil in preheated oven until salmon flakes easily with a fork, five to seven minutes per side.

SHRIMP

GARLIC BASIL GRILLED SHRIMP

Total Time: 21 min
Prep: 15 min
Cook: 6 min

8 Servings
2 Nutrient-Dense Protein Per Serving
2 Whole-Food Fat Per Serving

Ingredients

- 4 cloves garlic, minced
- 1/4 cup and 3 tablespoons extra virgin coconut oil
- 1/3 cup tomato sauce
- 2 tablespoons and 2 teaspoons red wine vinegar
- 2 tablespoons and 2 teaspoons chopped fresh basil
- 3/4 teaspoon salt
- 1/4 teaspoon cayenne pepper
- 2-3/4 pounds fresh shrimp, peeled and deveined
- skewers

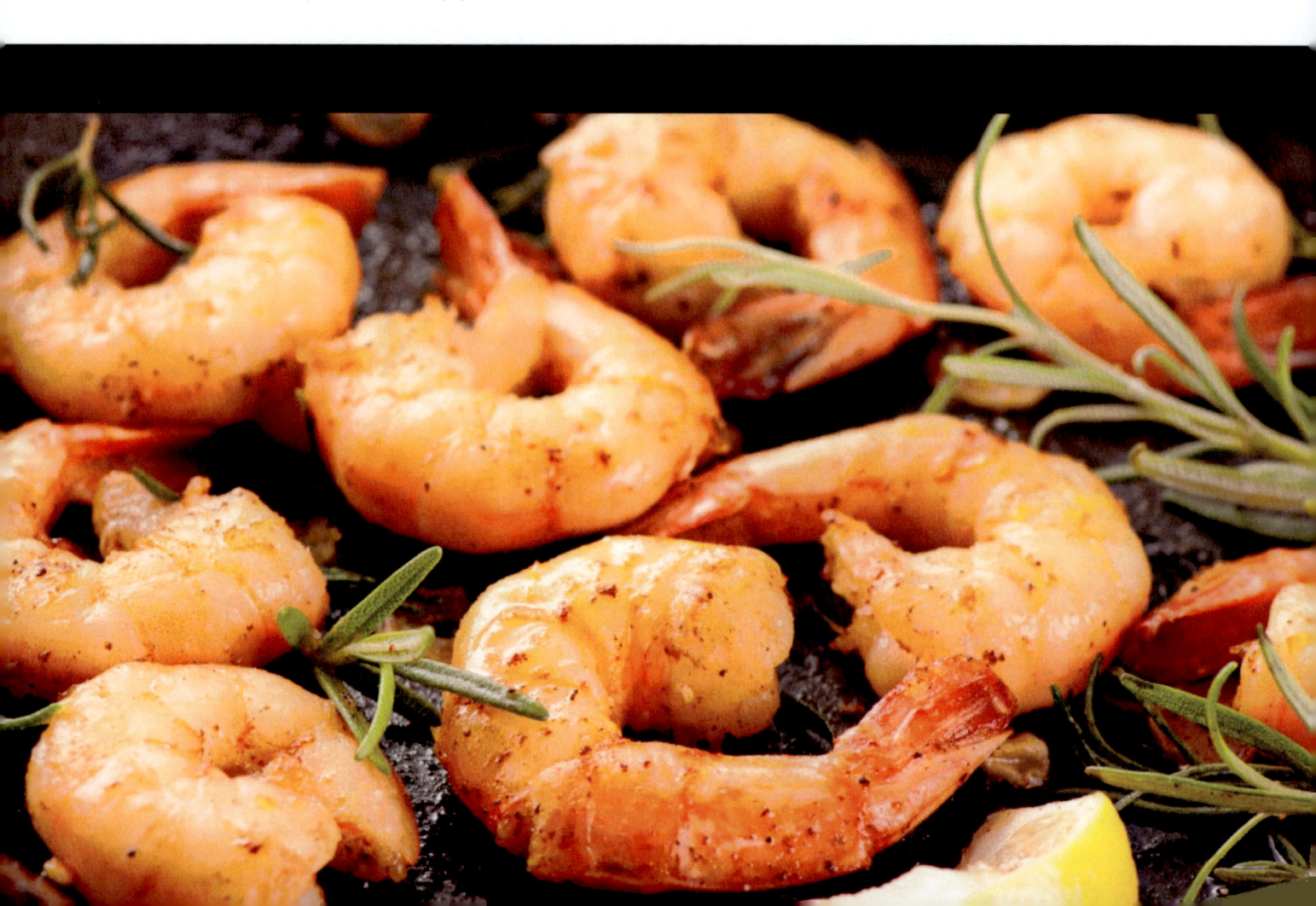

Directions

1. In a large bowl, stir together the garlic, coconut oil, tomato sauce, and red wine vinegar. Season with basil, salt, and cayenne pepper. Add shrimp to the bowl, and stir until evenly coated. Cover, and refrigerate for 30 minutes to 1 hour, stirring once or twice.

2. Preheat grill for medium heat. Thread shrimp onto skewers, piercing once near the tail and once near the head. Discard marinade.

3. Lightly oil grill grate. Cook shrimp on preheated grill for 2 to 3 minutes per side, or until opaque.

SANE   Free Tools: SANESolution.com/Tools   Superfoods: store.SANESolution.com

Italian Shrimp

Total Time: 45 min
Prep: 15 min
Cook: 30 min

8 Servings
1 Nutrient-Dense Protein Per Serving
1 Whole-Food Fat Per Serving

Ingredients

- 4 cloves garlic, minced
- 2 tablespoons and 2 teaspoons extra virgin coconut oil
- 1/3 cup tomato sauce
- 2 tablespoons and 2 teaspoons red wine vinegar
- 2 tablespoons and 2 teaspoons chopped fresh basil
- 3/4 teaspoon salt
- 1/4 teaspoon cayenne pepper
- 2-3/4 pounds fresh shrimp, peeled and deveined

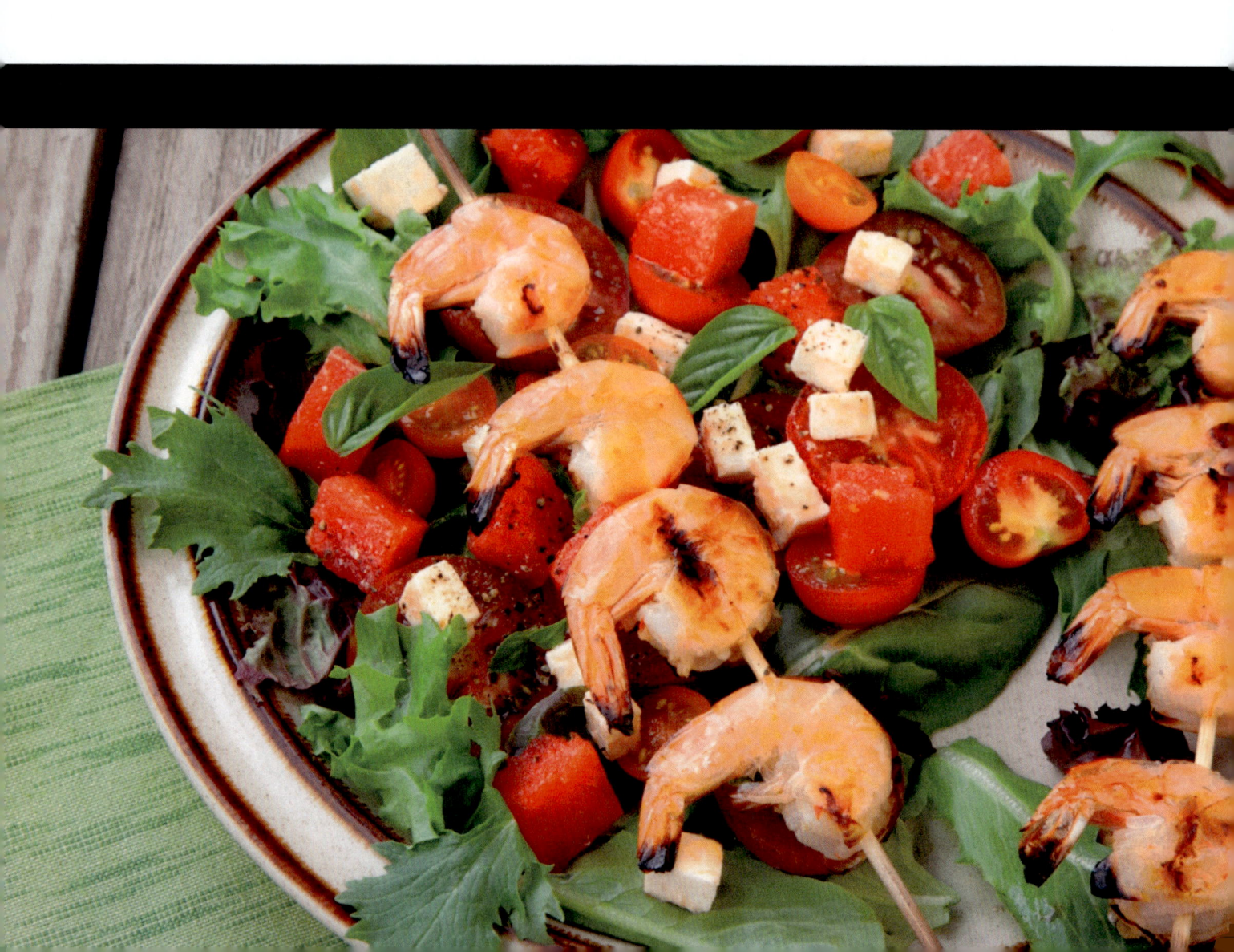

Directions

1. Stir garlic, melted extra virgin coconut oil, tomato sauce, and red wine vinegar in a large bowl. Season with basil, salt, and cayenne pepper. Add shrimp to the bowl and stir until evenly coated. Cover and refrigerate for 30 minutes to 1 hour, stirring once or twice.

2. Preheat grill for medium heat and lightly oil the grate.

3. Thread shrimp onto skewers, piercing once near tail and once near head. Discard marinade.

4. Cook shrimp on preheated grill until opaque, 2 to 3 minutes per side.

SANE Free Tools: SANESolution.com/Tools   Superfoods: store.SANESolution.com

Herbed Shrimp Scampi

Total Time: 20 min
Prep: 10 min
Cook: 10 min

8 Servings
2 Nutrient-Dense Protein Per Serving
3 Whole-Food Fat Per Serving

Ingredients

- 1-1/3 cups butter
- 1-1/4 cloves garlic, minced
- 1/4 teaspoon dried rosemary
- 1/4 teaspoon dried basil
- 1/4 cup lemon juice
- 2 tablespoons and 2 teaspoons dry white wine
- 3/4 teaspoon salt
- 3/4 teaspoon ground black pepper
- 2-3/4 pounds medium shrimp, peeled and deveined
- 6 12×12-inch squares of aluminum foil

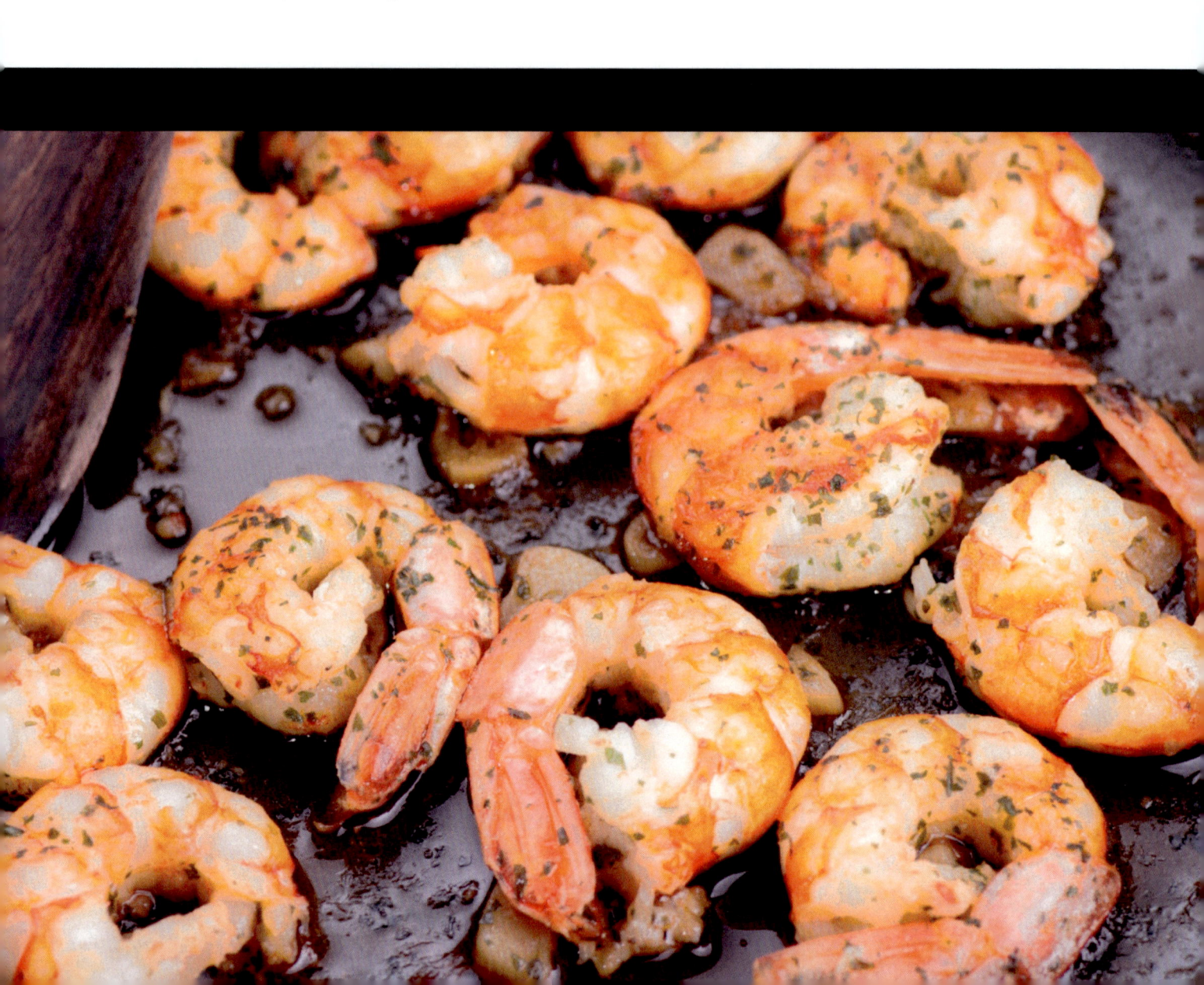

Directions

1. Preheat grill for medium heat.

2. Melt butter in a large skillet over medium heat; cook and stir garlic, rosemary, and basil in the hot butter until garlic is fragrant and beginning to brown, about 5 minutes. Stir lemon juice, white wine, salt, and black pepper into butter and garlic.

3. Arrange about 6 shrimp onto each square of aluminum foil and drizzle the butter and herb mixture over shrimp. Gather up the corners of the foil squares and twist the tops to form tight packets.

4. Grill the packets on the preheated grill until shrimp are opaque and pink, 10 to 12 minutes.

SANE

Free Tools: SANESolution.com/Tools   Superfoods: store.SANESolution.com

SPICED SHRIMP

Total Time: 21 min
Prep: 15 min
Cook: 6 min

8 Servings
1 Nutrient-Dense Protein Per Serving
1 Whole-Food Fat Per Serving

Ingredients

- 1-1/4 large cloves garlic
- 1 tablespoon and 1 teaspoon coarse salt
- 3/4 teaspoon cayenne pepper
- 1-1/4 teaspoons paprika
- 2 tablespoons and 2 teaspoons extra virgin coconut oil
- 2-3/4 teaspoons lemon juice
- 2-3/4 pounds large shrimp, peeled and deveined
- 10-1/2 wedges lemon, for garnish

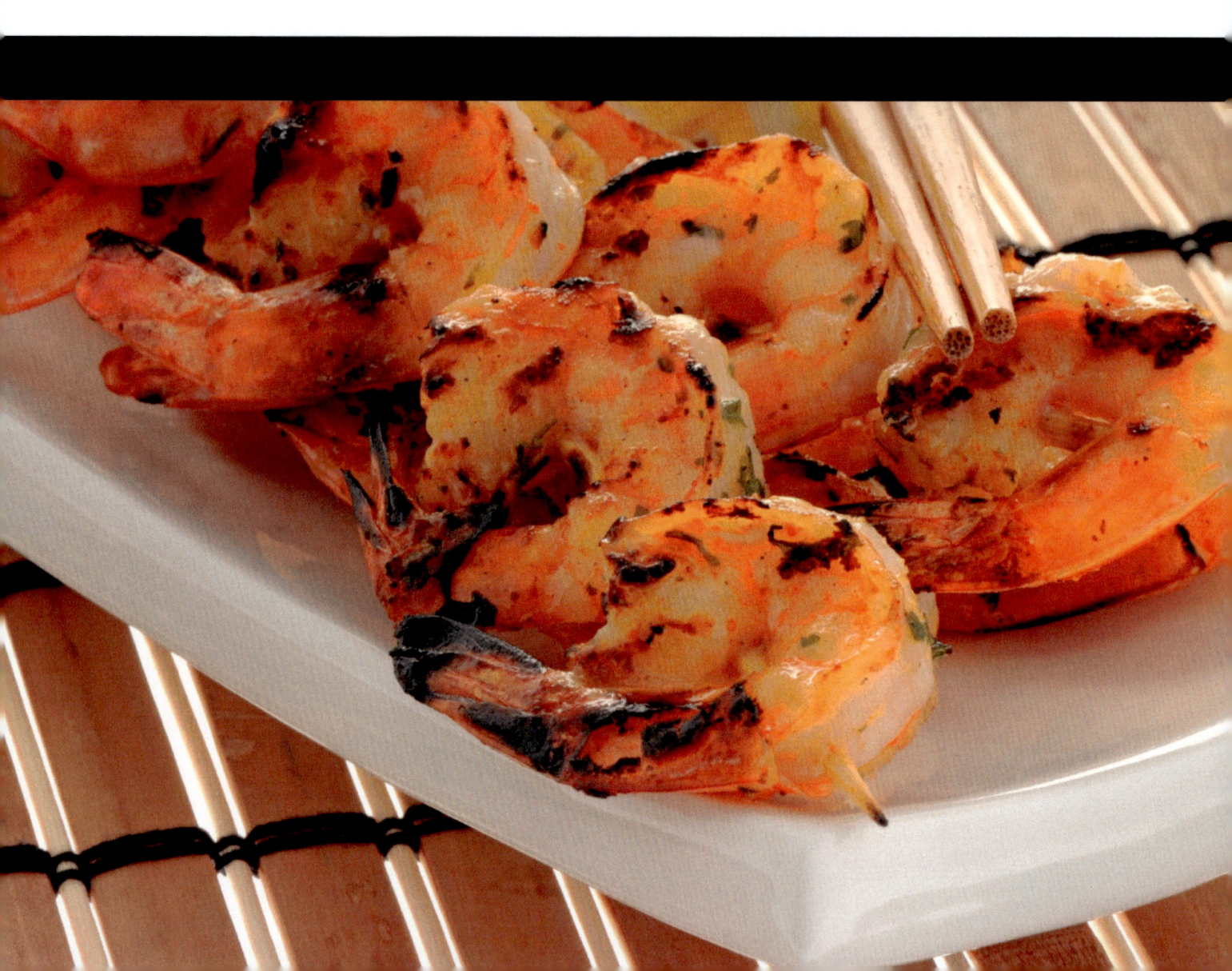

Directions

1. Preheat grill for medium heat.

2. In a small bowl, crush the garlic with the salt. Mix in cayenne pepper and paprika, and then stir in olive oil and lemon juice to form a paste. In a large bowl, toss shrimp with garlic paste until evenly coated.

3. Lightly oil grill grate. Cook shrimp for 2 to 3 minutes per side, or until opaque. Transfer to a serving dish, garnish with lemon wedges, and serve..

Shrimp Basil

Total Time: 30 min
Prep: 25 min
Cook: 5 min

8 Servings
1 Nutrient-Dense Protein Per Serving
1 Whole-Food Fat Per Serving

Ingredients

- 3 tablespoons
- 4 tablespoons butter, melted
- 1-1/4 lemons, juiced
- 2 tablespoons and 2 teaspoons Dijon mustard
- 1/4 cup and 3 tablespoons minced fresh basil leaves
- 2-3/4 cloves garlic, minced
- salt to taste
- white pepper
- 2-3/4 pounds fresh shrimp, peeled and deveined
- skewers

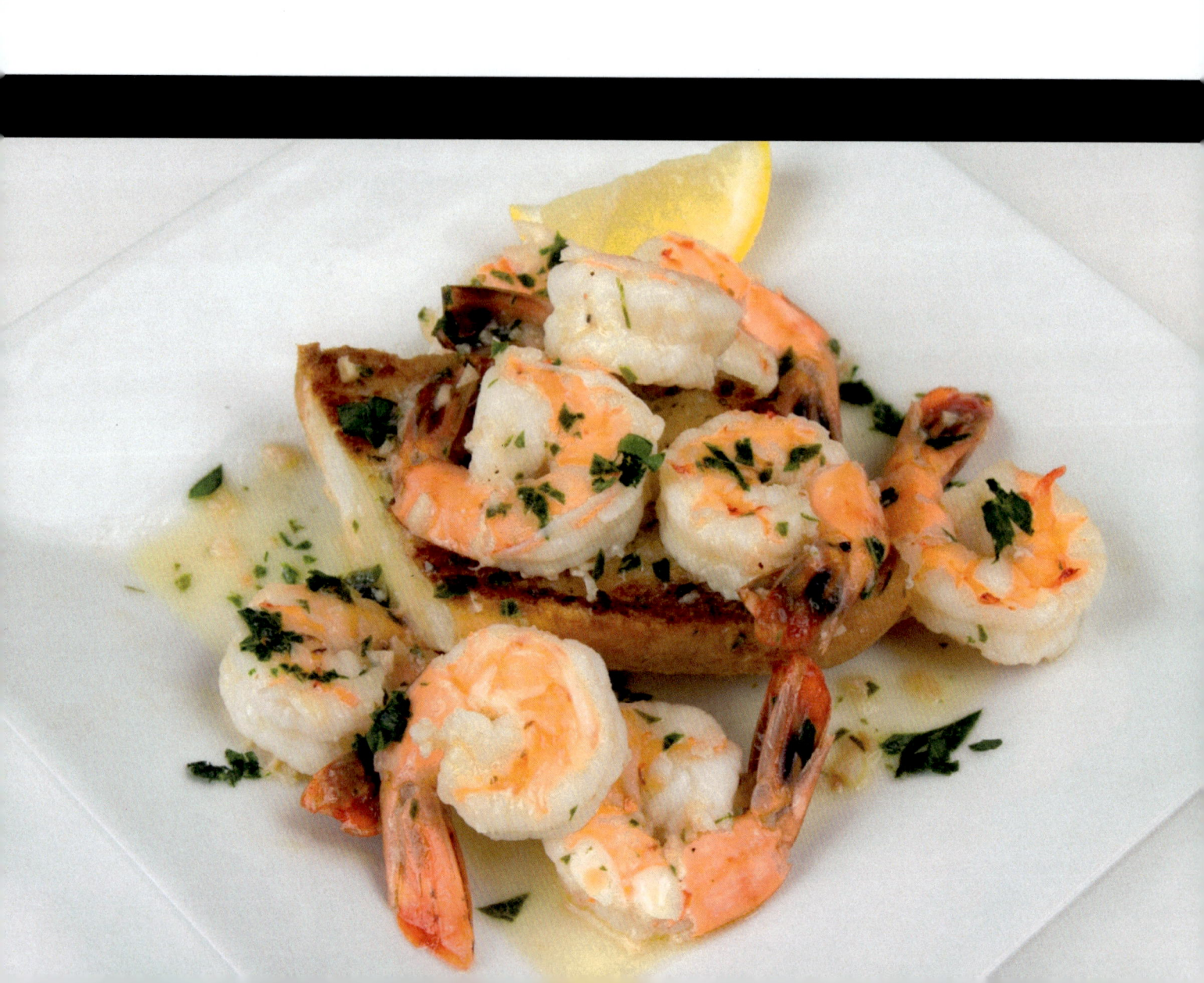

Directions

1. In a shallow, non-porous dish or bowl, mix together melted extra virgin coconut oil and melted butter. Stir in lemon juice, mustard, basil, and garlic, and season with salt and white pepper. Add shrimp, and toss to coat. Cover, and refrigerate for 1 hour.

2. Preheat grill to high heat. Remove shrimp from marinade, and thread onto skewers. Discard marinade.

3. Lightly oil grill grate, and arrange skewers on preheated grill. Cook for 4 minutes, turning once, or until opaque.

SANE Free Tools: SANESolution.com/Tools   Superfoods: store.SANESolution.com

Bayou Shrimp

Total Time: 10 min
Prep: 5 min
Cook: 5 min

8 Servings
1 Nutrient-Dense Protein Per Serving
1 Whole-Food Fat Per Serving

Ingredients

- 2 teaspoons paprika
- 1-1/2 teaspoons dried thyme
- 1-1/2 teaspoons dried oregano
- 1/2 teaspoon garlic powder
- 1/2 teaspoon salt
- 1/2 teaspoon ground black pepper
- 1/2 teaspoon cayenne pepper, or more to taste
- 3 pounds large shrimp, peeled and deveined
- 2 tablespoons extra virgin coconut oil

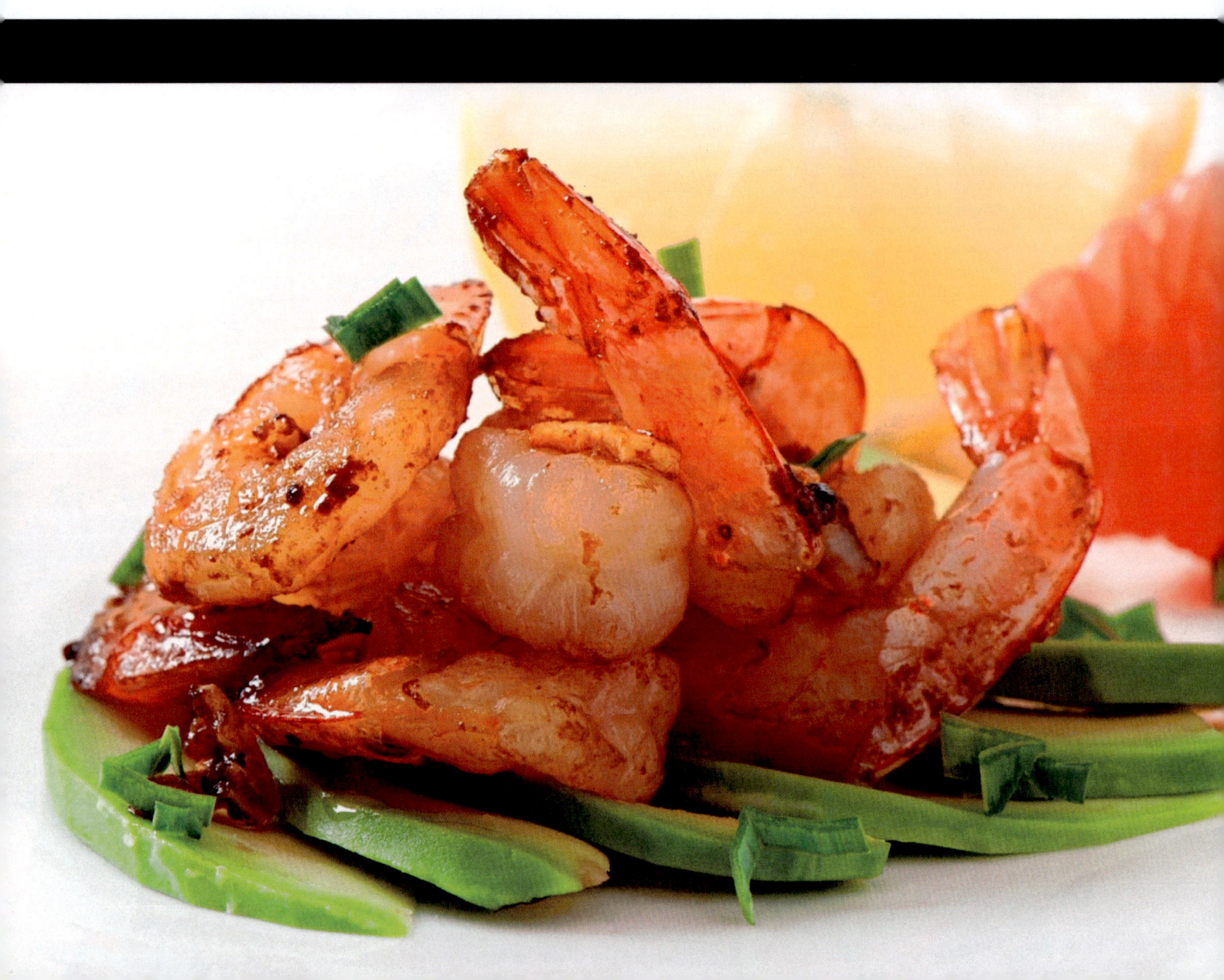

Directions

1. Combine paprika, thyme, oregano, garlic powder, salt, pepper, and cayenne pepper in a sealable plastic bag; shake to mix. Add shrimp and shake to coat.

2. Heat oil in a large non-stick skillet over medium high heat. Cook and stir shrimp in hot oil until they are bright pink on the outside and the meat is no longer transparent in the center, about 4 minutes.

SANE Free Tools: SANESolution.com/Tools   Superfoods: store.SANESolution.com

Tilapia

Old Bay Tilapia

Total Time: 35 min
Prep: 5 min
Cook: 30 min

8 Servings
1 Nutrient-Dense Protein Per Serving
1 Whole-Food Fat Per Serving

Ingredients

- 8 (4 ounce) fillets tilapia
- 1 tablespoon and 1 teaspoon butter
- 1/2 teaspoon seafood seasoning
- 1 teaspoon garlic salt, or to taste
- 2 lemon, sliced
- 2 (16 ounce) packages frozen cauliflower with broccoli and red pepper

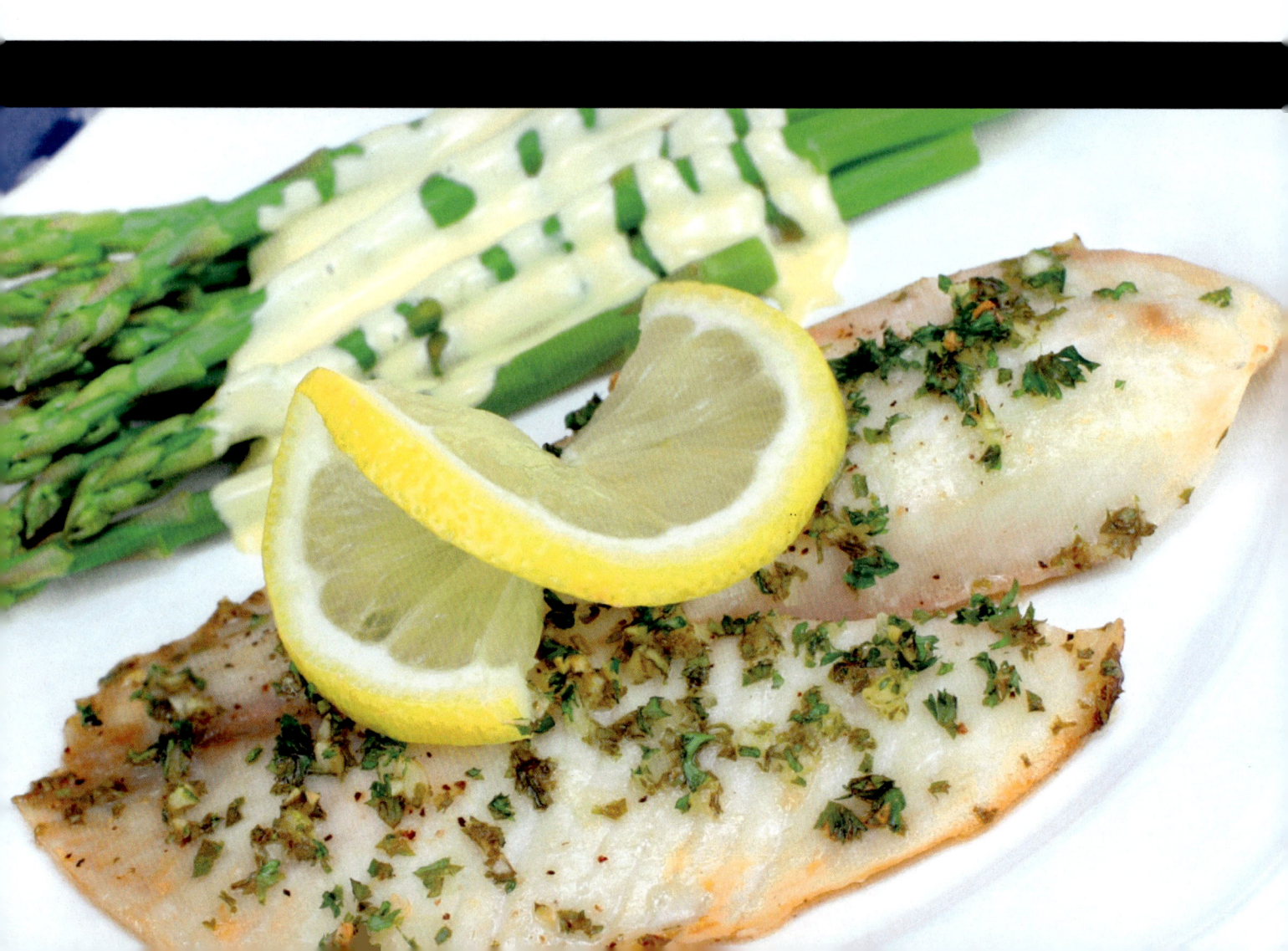

Directions

1. Preheat the oven to 375 degrees F (190 degrees F). Grease a 9×13 inch baking dish.

2. Place the tilapia fillets in the bottom of the baking dish and dot with butter. Season with seafood seasoning and garlic salt. Top each one with a slice or two of lemon. Arrange the frozen mixed vegetables around the fish, and season lightly with salt and pepper.

3. Cover the dish and bake for 25 to 30 minutes in the preheated oven, until vegetables are tender and fish flakes easily with a fork.

Mustard Tilapia

Total Time: 20 min
Prep: 5 min
Cook: 15 min

8 Servings
2 Nutrient-Dense Protein Per Serving
1 Whole-Food Fat Per Serving

Ingredients

- 8 (6 ounce) fresh tilapia fillets
- 1 tablespoon and 1 teaspoon spicy brown mustard
- 1 tablespoon and 1 teaspoon Worcestershire sauce
- 2 teaspoons lemon juice
- 1 teaspoon garlic powder
- 1 teaspoon dried oregano
- 2 teaspoons grated Parmesan cheese
- 1 tablespoon and 1 teaspoon fine Italian bread

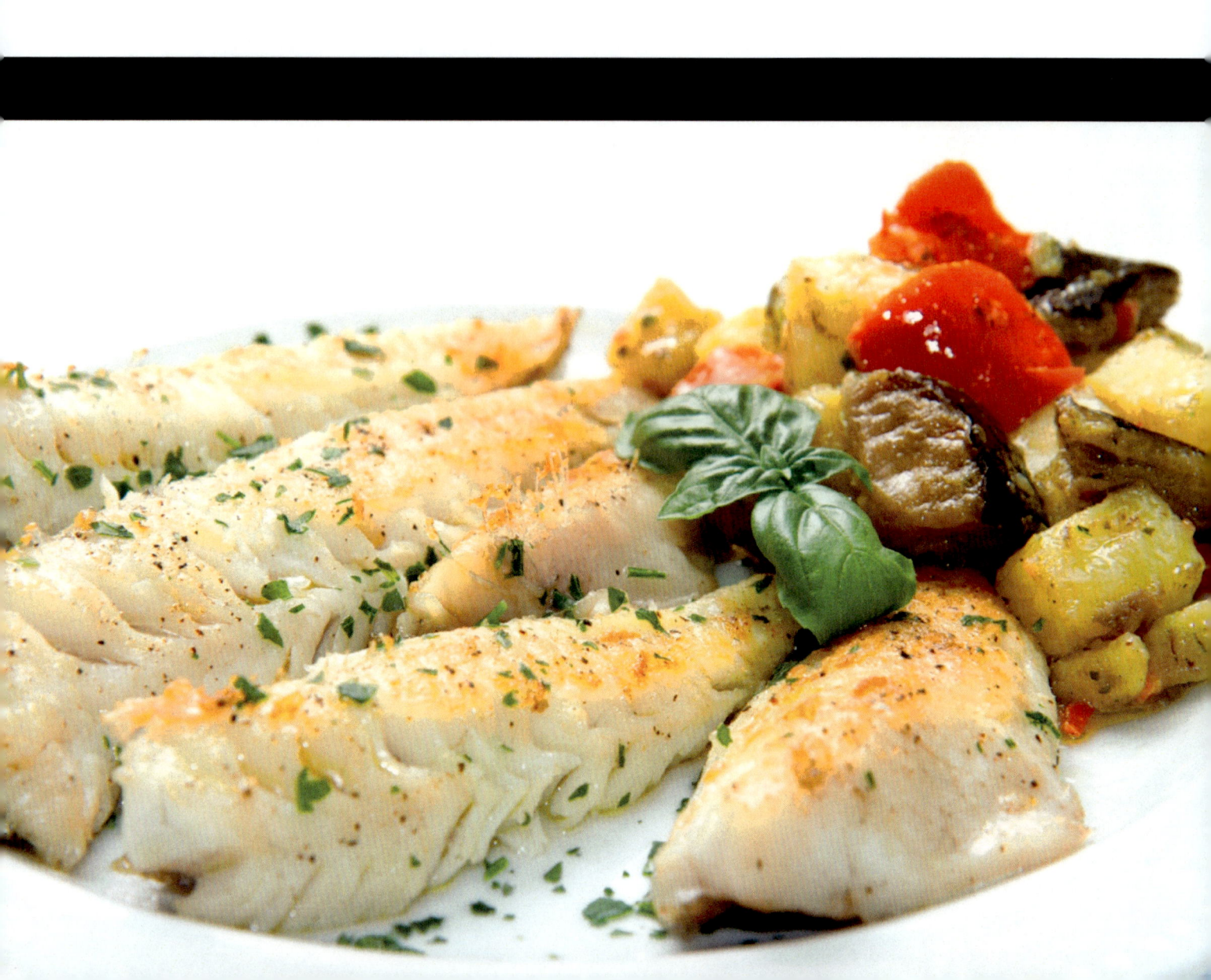

Directions

1. Preheat oven to 375 degrees F (190 degrees C). Spray a glass baking dish with cooking spray.

2. Place tilapia fillets into prepared baking dish, and bake in preheated oven for 10 minutes. Meanwhile, stir together the mustard, Worcestershire sauce, lemon juice, garlic powder, oregano, and Parmesan cheese.

3. When fish has cooked for 10 minutes, spread with herb paste, and sprinkle with bread crumbs. Continue baking for another 5 minutes until the topping is bubbly and golden.

SANE Free Tools: SANESolution.com/Tools   Superfoods: store.SANESolution.com

Tahini Fish

Total Time: 1hr
Prep: 15 min
Cook: 45 min

8 Servings
1 Nutrient-Dense Protein Per Serving
2 Whole-Food Fat Per Serving

Ingredients

- 3 pounds catfish fillets
- 2/3 cup tahini
- 4 cloves garlic, minced
- 1/2 cup water
- 1/2 cup fresh lemon juice
- salt to taste
- 2 tablespoons chopped fresh parsley

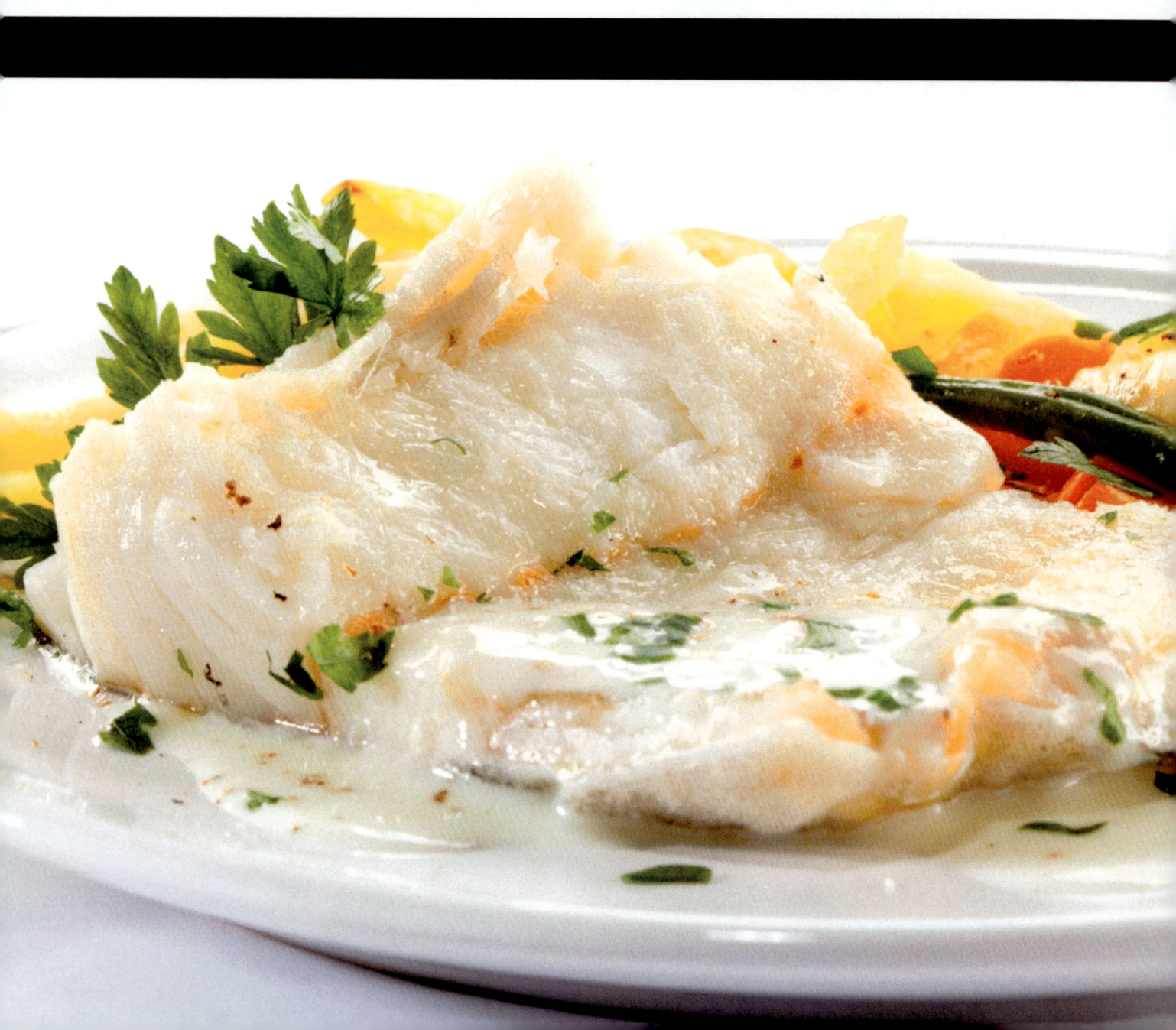

Directions

1. Preheat an oven to 375 degrees F (190 degrees C). Grease a baking dish and arrange the catfish in a single layer.

2. Bake in the preheated oven until the fish flakes easily with a fork, 45 to 60 minutes.

3. Meanwhile, whisk together the tahini, garlic, water, and lemon juice; season with salt. Once the fish is done, cut it into 1 inch cubes, and pour the tahini sauce overtop. Sprinkle with parsley to garnish.

SANE Free Tools: SANESolution.com/Tools   Superfoods: store.SANESolution.com

Parmesan Tilapia

Total Time: 15 min
Prep: 5 min
Cook: 10 min

8 Servings
1 Nutrient-Dense Protein Per Serving
1 Whole-Food Fat Per Serving

Ingredients

- 1/2 cup Parmesan cheese
- 1/8 cup butter, softened
- 3 tablespoons light mayonnaise
- 2 tablespoons fresh lemon juice
- 1/4 teaspoon dried basil
- 1/4 teaspoon ground black pepper
- 1/8 teaspoon onion powder
- 1/8 teaspoon celery salt
- 2 pounds tilapia fillets

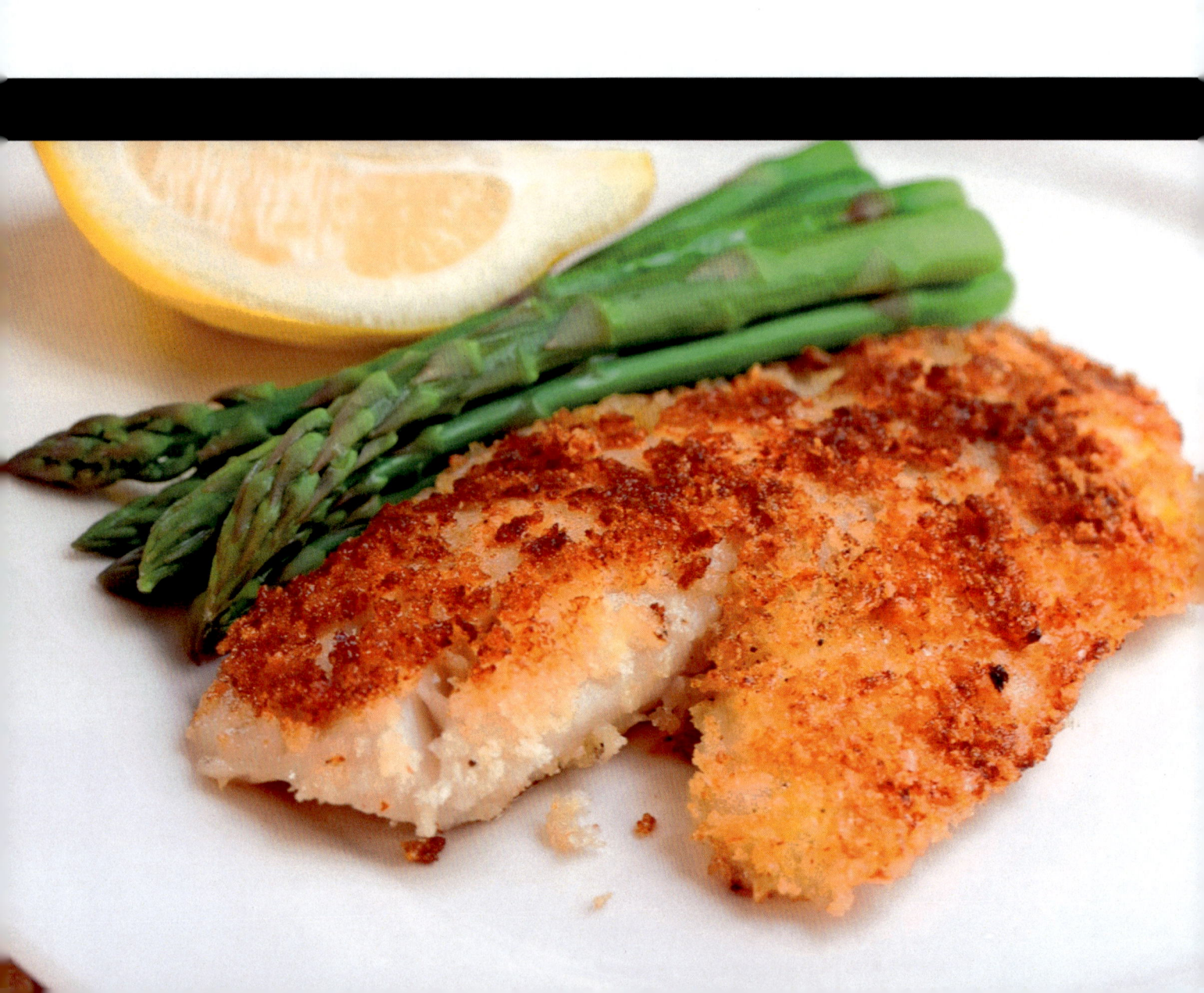

Directions

1. Preheat oven broiler. Grease broiling pan or line with aluminum foil.

2. Mix Parmesan cheese, butter, mayonnaise, and lemon juice together in a small bowl. Season with dried basil, pepper, onion powder, and celery salt. Mix well and set aside. Arrange fillets in a single layer on prepared pan.

3. Broil a few inches from the heat for 2 to 3 minutes. Flip fillets over and broil for 2 or 3 minutes more. Remove fillets from oven and cover with Parmesan mixture on top side. Broil until fish flakes easily with a fork, about 2 minutes.

Tilapia Feta Florentine

Total Time: 55 min
Prep: 20 min
Cook: 35 min

8 Servings
1 Nutrient-Dense Protein Per Serving
1 Whole-Food Fat Per Serving

Ingredients

- 1 tablespoon and 1 teaspoon extra virgin coconut oil
- 1/2 cup chopped onion
- 2 cloves garlic, minced
- 4 (9 ounce) bags fresh spinach
- 1/2 cup sliced kalamata olives
- 1/4 cup crumbled feta cheese
- 1 teaspoon grated lemon rind
- 1 teaspoon salt
- 1/2 teaspoon dried oregano
- 1/4 teaspoon white pepper
- 2 pounds tilapia fillets
- 1/4 cup butter, melted
- 1 tablespoon and 1 teaspoon lemon juice
- 2 pinches paprika, or to taste

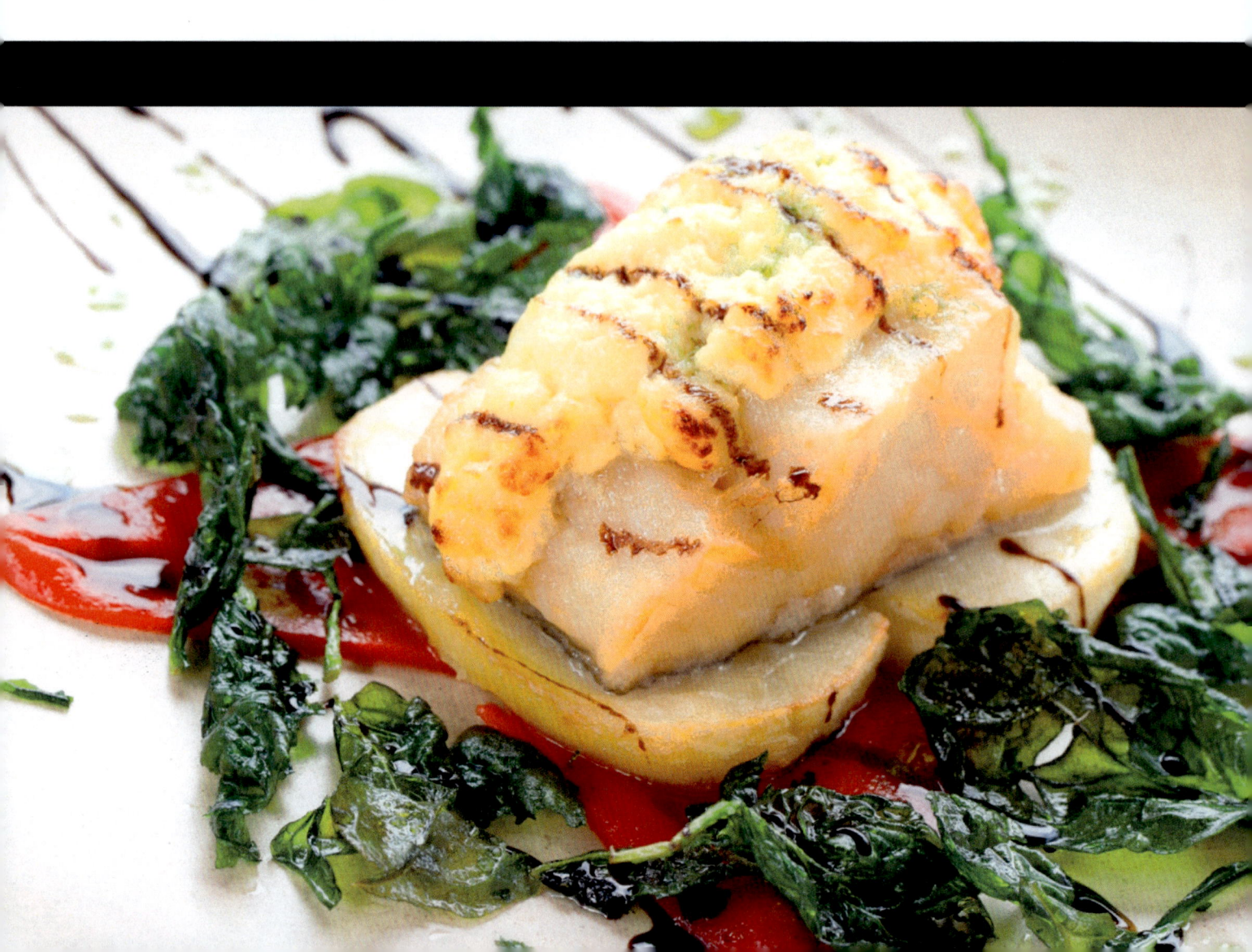

Directions

1. Preheat oven to 400 degrees F (200 degrees C).

2. Heat extra virgin coconut oil in a large skillet over medium heat; cook and stir onion and garlic in the hot oil until onion is soft, about 5 minutes. Add spinach to skillet; cook and stir until spinach is wilted and cooked down, 5 more minutes. Stir olives, feta cheese, lemon rind, salt, oregano, and white pepper into spinach. Cook until feta cheese has melted and flavors have blended, about 5 more minutes.

3. Spread spinach mixture into a 9×13-inch baking dish. Arrange tilapia fillets over spinach mixture. Mix butter and lemon juice in a small bowl and drizzle over fish; sprinkle with paprika.

4. Bake fish in the preheated oven until the flesh is opaque and flakes easily, 20 to 25 minutes.

SANE Free Tools: SANESolution.com/Tools   Superfoods: store.SANESolution.com

Delicate Parmesan Tilapia

Total Time: 15 min
Prep: 5 min
Cook: 10 min

8 Servings
1 Nutrient-Dense Protein Per Serving
1 Whole-Food Fat Per Serving

Ingredients

- 1/2 cup Parmesan cheese
- 1/4 cup butter, softened
- 3 tablespoons mayonnaise
- 2 tablespoons fresh lemon juice
- 1/4 teaspoon dried basil
- 1/4 teaspoon ground black pepper
- 1/8 teaspoon onion powder
- 1/8 teaspoon celery salt
- 2 pounds tilapia fillets

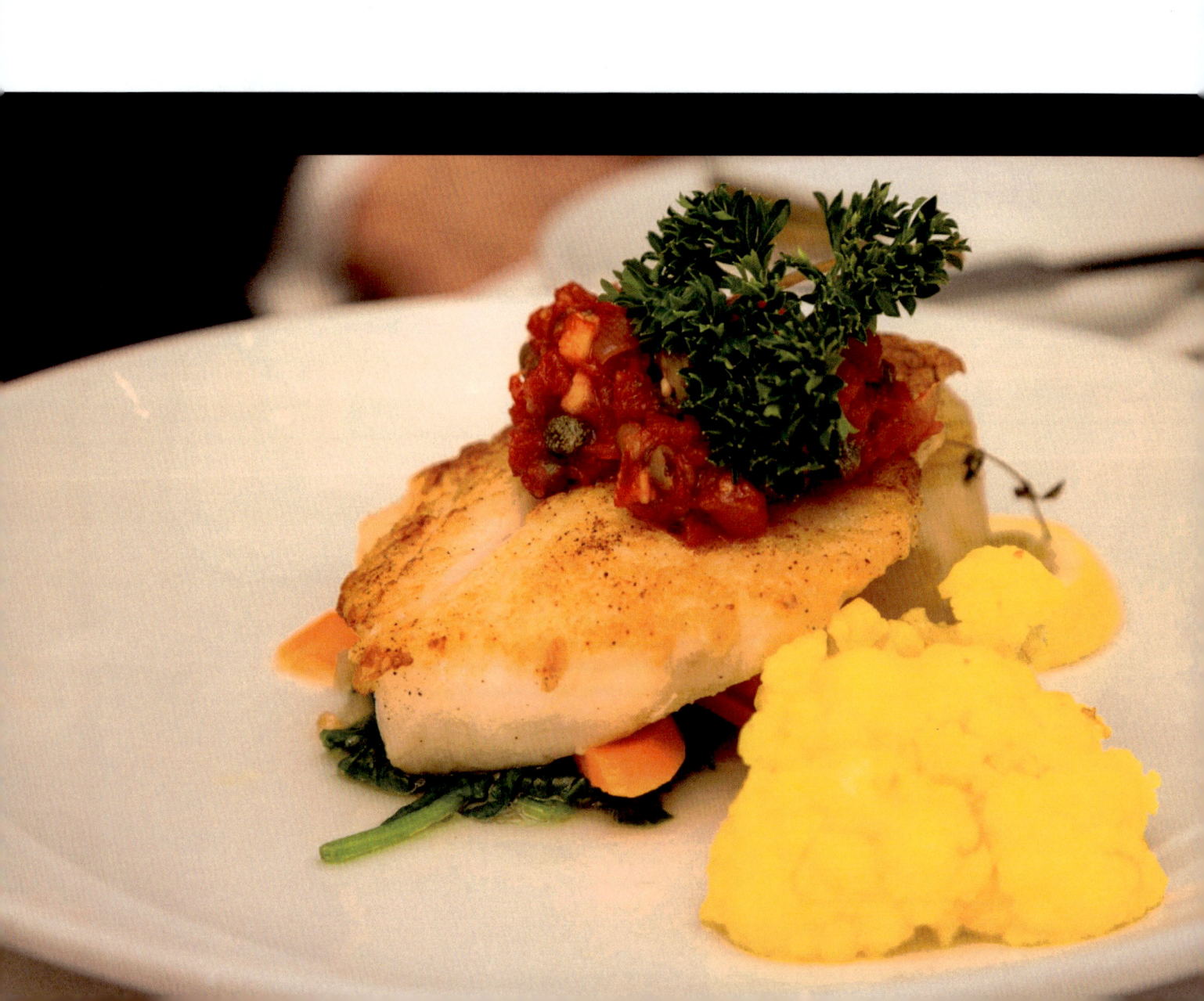

Directions

1. Preheat your oven's broiler. Grease a broiling pan or line pan with aluminum foil.

2. In a small bowl, mix together the Parmesan cheese, butter, mayonnaise and lemon juice. Season with dried basil, pepper, onion powder and celery salt. Mix well and set aside.

3. Arrange fillets in a single layer on the prepared pan. Broil a few inches from the heat for 2 to 3 minutes. Flip the fillets over and broil for a couple more minutes. Remove the fillets from the oven and cover them with the Parmesan cheese mixture on the top side. Broil for 2 more minutes or until the topping is browned and fish flakes easily with a fork. Be careful not to over cook the fish.

SANE — Free Tools: SANESolution.com/Tools — Superfoods: store.SANESolution.com

Trout

Bacon Trout

Total Time: 50 min
Prep: 25 min
Cook: 25 min

8 Servings
1 Nutrient-Dense Protein Per Serving
1 Whole-Food Fat Per Serving

Ingredients

- 1/2 cup butter
- 2 lemon, juiced
- 1/4 cup seeded and diced jalapeno pepper
- 1/4 cup diced green onion
- 1 clove garlic, minced
- sea salt and ground black pepper to taste
- 4 (10 ounce) cleaned whole trout, heads removed
- 4 sprigs fresh dill
- 4 slices bacon

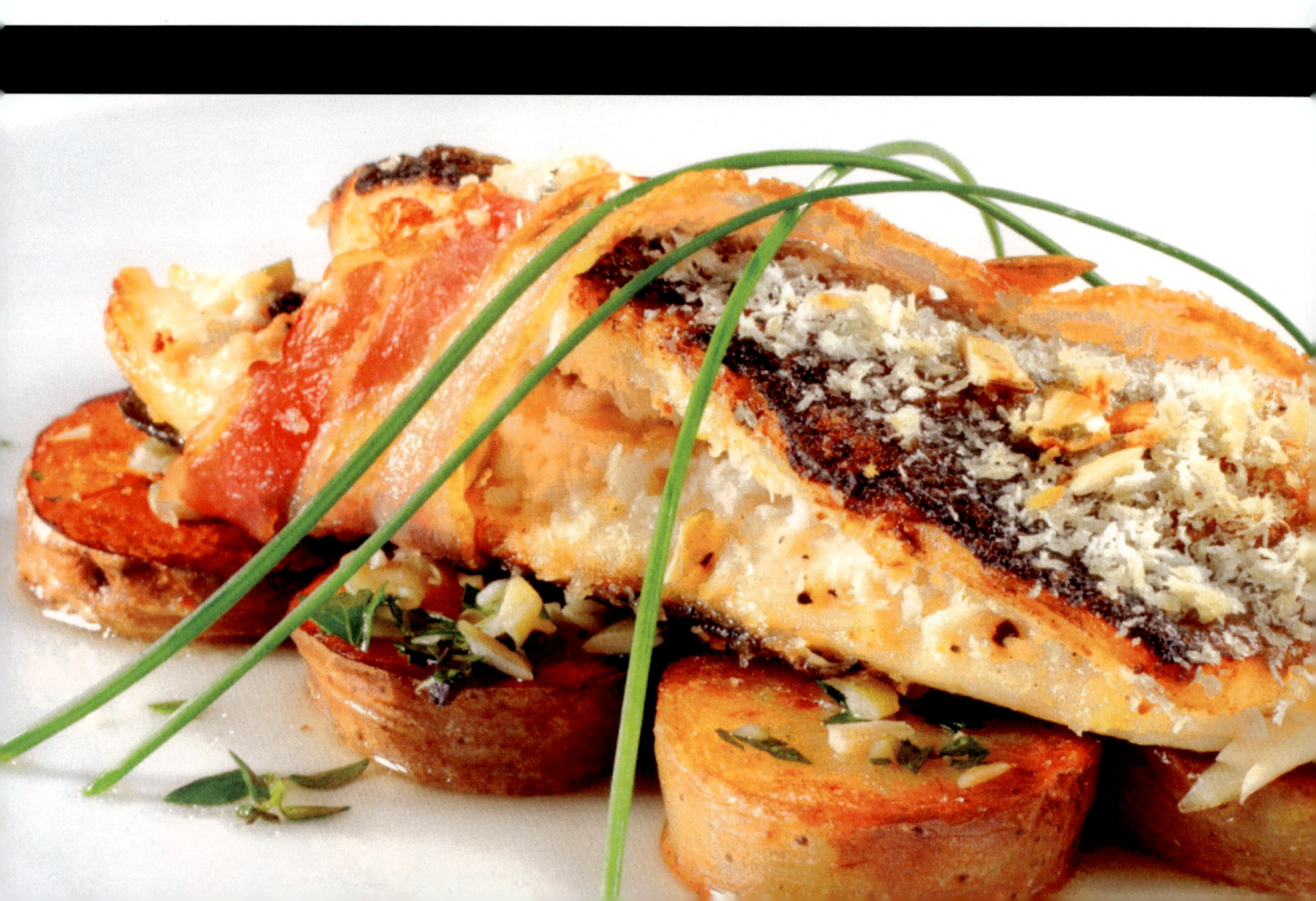

Directions

1. Preheat oven to 400 degrees F (200 degrees C). Line a 9×13-inch glass baking dish with foil.

2. Place a small saucepan over low heat; heat butter until partially melted. Stir in lemon juice, jalapeno pepper, green onion, and garlic; stir mixture into a paste. Season with sea salt and black pepper.

3. Place each trout onto a large sheet of aluminum foil and stuff the cavity of each fish with butter paste; place a dill sprig and a bacon strip into the cavity over the butter mixture. Fold foil over fish and wrap edges to seal tightly. Place foil packets in the prepared baking dish.

4. Bake foil packets until fish flakes easily with a fork, 26 minutes. Let fish sit in foil packet for 5 minutes before unwrapping. To serve, transfer fish from foil to a serving plate; discard bacon. Flesh of fish will be white and skin will peel off.

Mango Trout

Total Time: 50 min
Prep: 30 min
Cook: 20 min

8 Servings
2 Nutrient-Dense Protein Per Serving
1 Whole-Food Fat Per Serving

Ingredients

- 4 whole trout, cleaned
- 3 medium fresh jalapeno pepper, chopped
- 4 medium green onions, chopped
- 1 bunch cilantro, chopped
- 1/2 cup bell pepper, diced
- 1/2 cup peeled, diced ripe mango
- 1/4 cup extra virgin coconut oil
- 2 tablespoons lime juice
- garlic salt to taste
- black pepper to taste

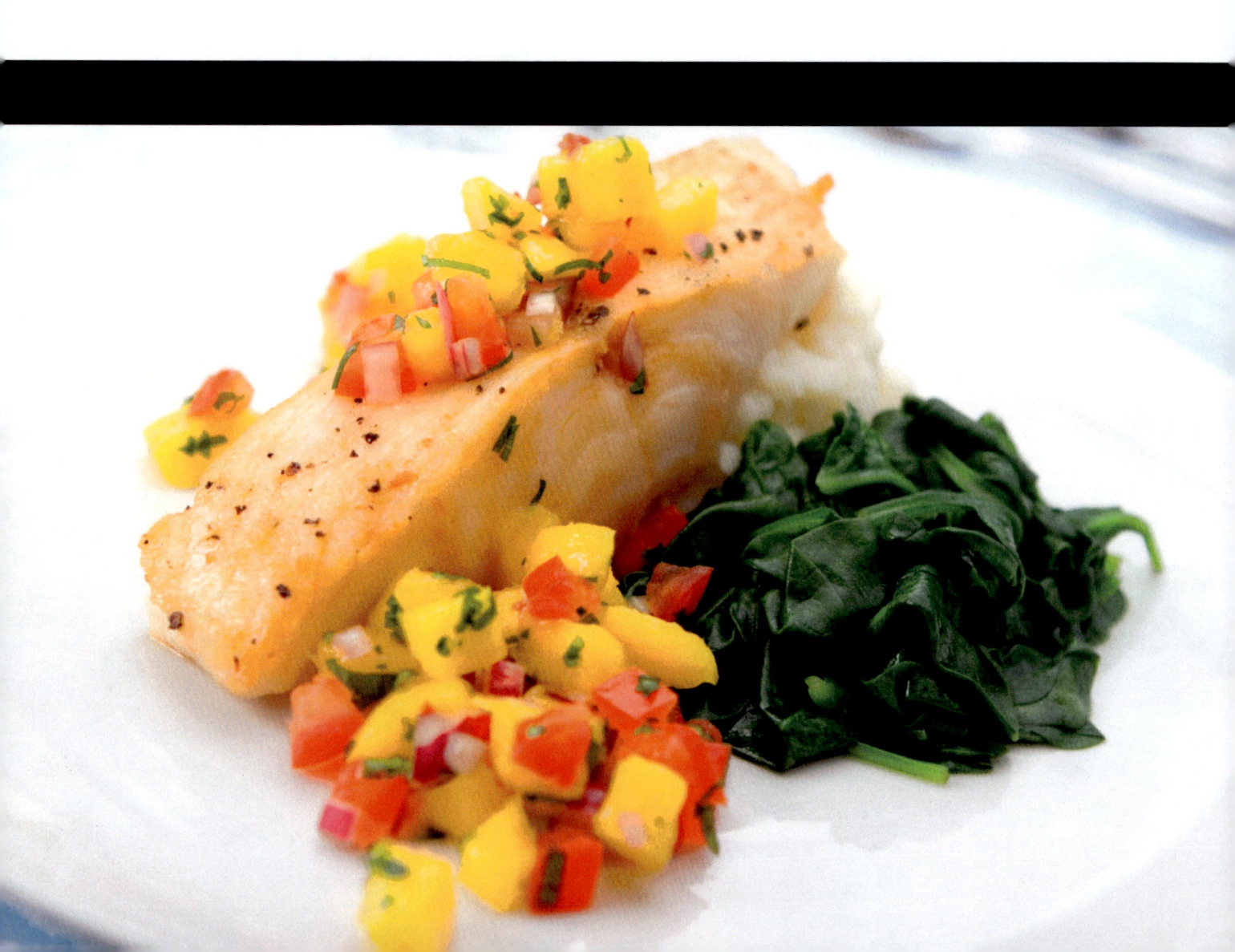

Directions

1. Preheat a grill for medium heat, and place the rack 3 inches over the coals.

2. In a medium bowl, mix together the green onions, cilantro, bell pepper, mango, melted extra virgin coconut oil, lime juice, garlic salt, and black pepper; set aside. Lightly coat four squares of foil with extra virgin coconut oil. Place fish diagonally on the foil, and stuff each with 1/4 of the mango stuffing. If it doesn't all fit inside the fish, then just place the remainder on top of the fish. Fold the corners of the foil over the head and tail of the fish, then fold the remaining corners over the body of the fish.

3. Cook the packets on both sides for about 20 minutes total, until the fish has cooked and flakes easily.

Italian Trout

Total Time: 50 min
Prep: 15 min
Cook: 35 min

8 Servings
2 Nutrient-Dense Protein Per Serving
1 Whole-Food Fat Per Serving

Ingredients

- 1 (4 pound) whole trout, cleaned
- salt and pepper to taste
- 1 (28 ounce) can diced tomatoes
- 2 tablespoons extra virgin coconut oil
- 2 tablespoons chopped fresh parsley
- 1 clove garlic, minced
- 1/2 cup white wine
- 1 lemon, cut into wedges
- 4 sprigs fresh parsley

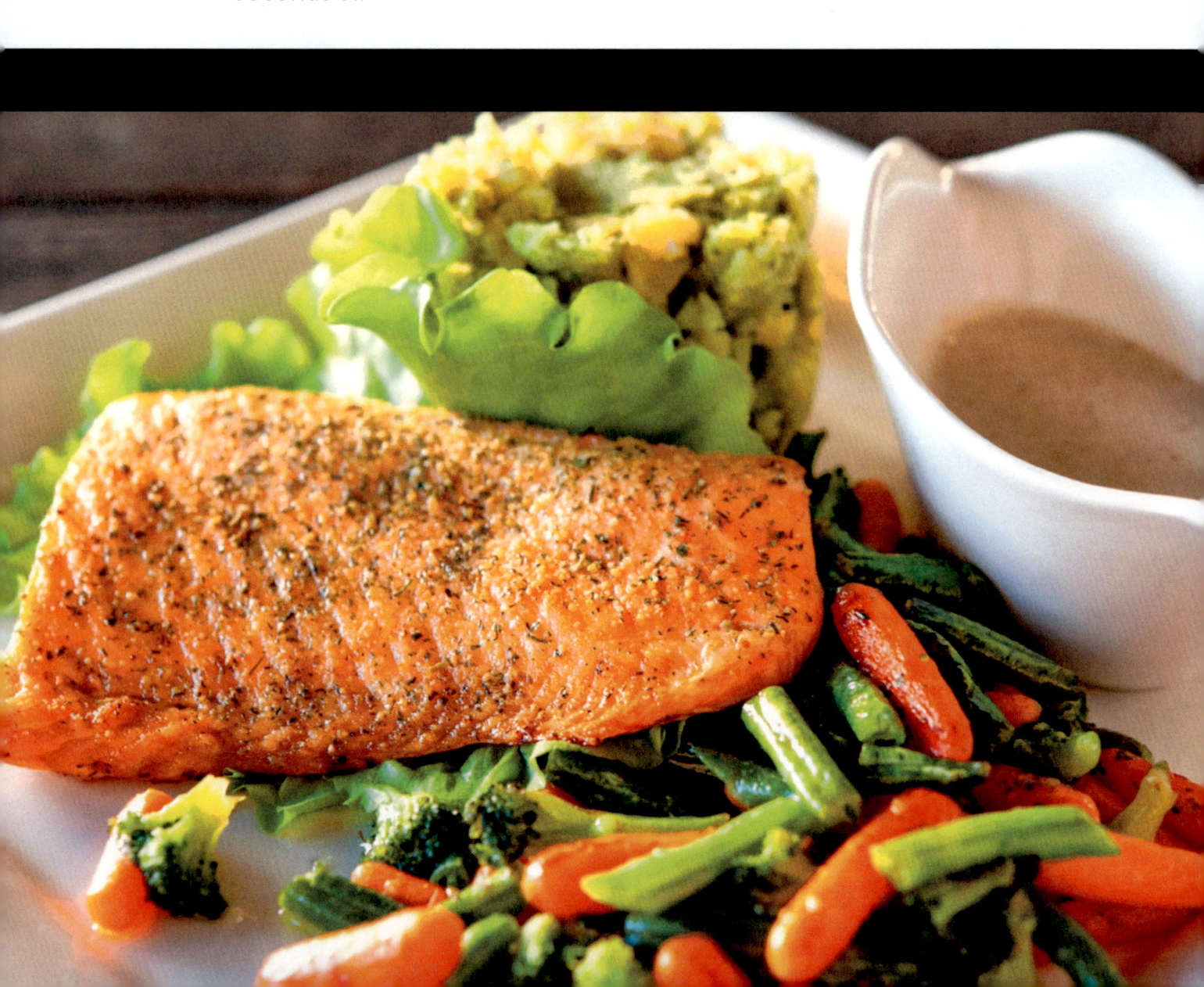

Directions

1. Preheat oven to 400 degrees F (205 degrees C). Lightly oil a 9×13 inch baking dish. Season the trout inside and out with salt and pepper to taste, and place in baking dish.

2. In a large bowl, combine tomatoes, melted coconut oil, 2 tablespoons chopped parsley, and minced garlic. Spread evenly over the fish.

3. Bake for 35 minutes, or until fish flakes easily. Baste during baking with wine. Serve garnished with lemon wedges and parsley sprigs.

Mushroom Trout

Total Time: 50 min
Prep: 15 min
Cook: 35 min

8 Servings
2 Nutrient-Dense Protein Per Serving
2 Whole-Food Fat Per Serving

Ingredients

- 2/3 cup butter
- 4 lemons, juiced
- 18-1/2 fresh mushrooms, sliced
- 1/3 cup sherry wine
- 4 pounds trout fillets
- salt to taste
- cracked black pepper to taste

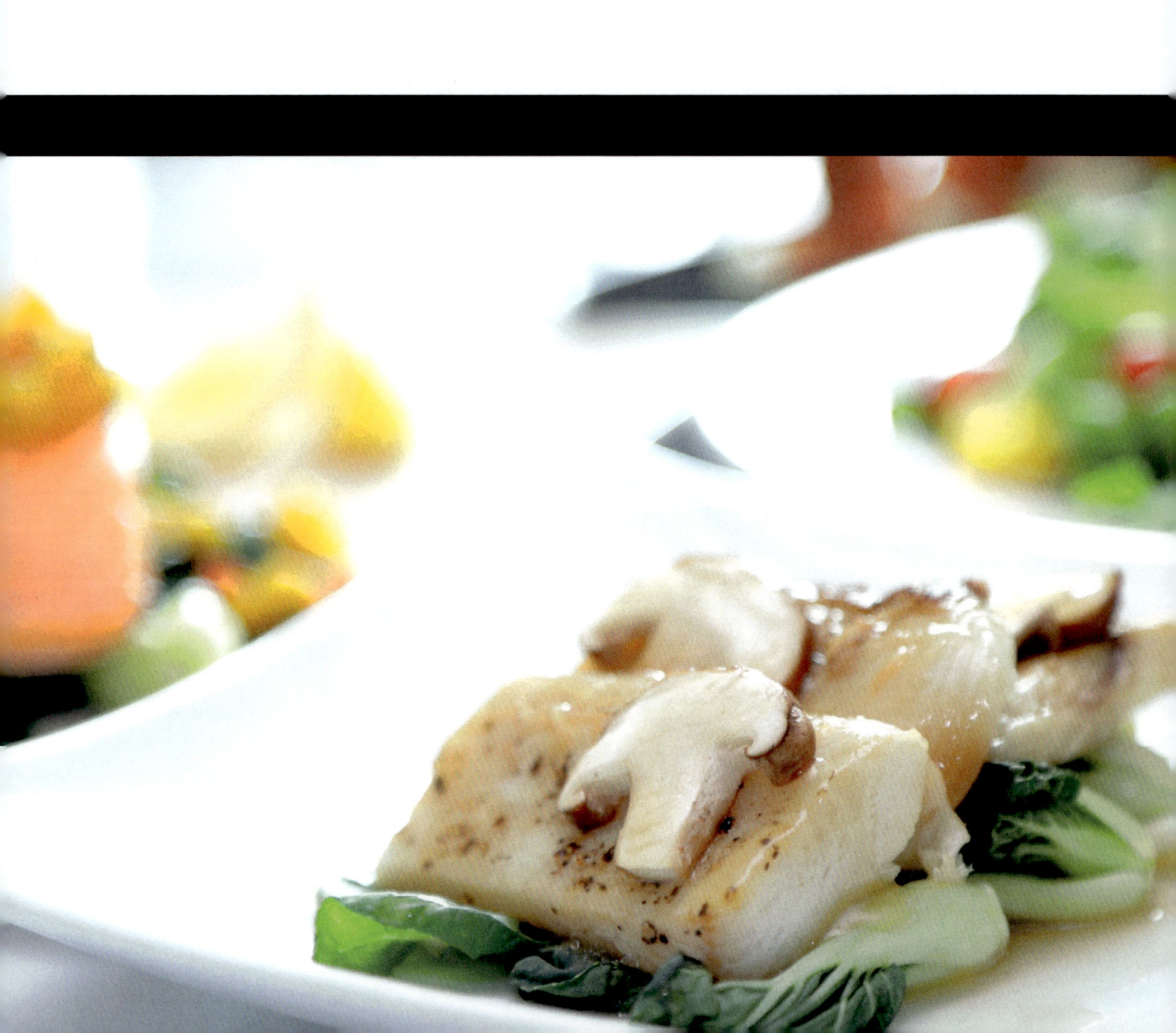

Directions

1. Preheat oven to 350 degrees F (175 degrees C). Line a shallow baking dish with foil.

2. Heat butter in a skillet over medium heat; pour in lemon juice. Cook and stir mushrooms until tender, about 5 minutes; stir in sherry. Place trout fillets with skin sides down into prepared baking dish; sprinkle with salt and cracked pepper. Pour the mushroom mixture over the fish.

3. Bake in the preheated oven until sauce reduces and fish flakes easily with a fork, about 30 minutes.

SANE   Free Tools: SANESolution.com/Tools   Superfoods: store.SANESolution.com

BBQ Trout

Total Time: 20 min
Prep: 10 min
Cook: 10 min

8 Servings
1 Nutrient-Dense Protein Per Serving
2 Whole-Food Fat Per Serving

Ingredients

- 2/3 cup soy sauce
- 2 tablespoons and 2 teaspoons extra virgin coconut oil
- 1-1/4 teaspoons dried rosemary
- 3/4 cup and 2 tablespoons and 1 teaspoon ketchup
- 2 tablespoons and 2 teaspoons lemon juice
- 8 (6 ounce) fillets rainbow trout

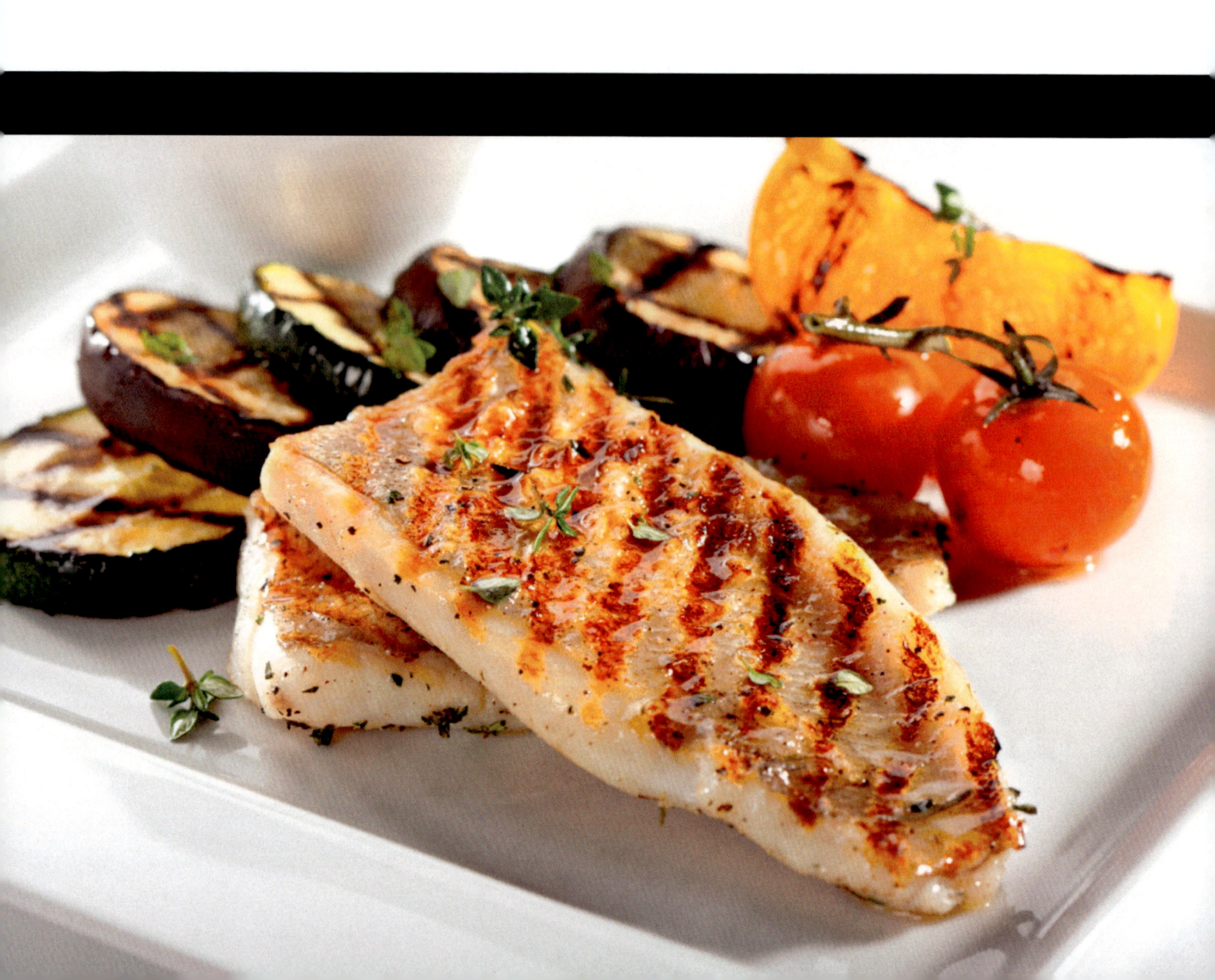

Directions

1. In a medium bowl, mix together soy sauce, extra virgin coconut oil, dried rosemary, ketchup and lemon juice. Set marinade aside.

2. Place rainbow trout in a medium baking dish, and pour marinade over the fish. Refrigerate for approximately 1 hour, turning trout once.

3. Preheat an outdoor grill for medium high heat and lightly oil grate. Drain excess marinade from fish, and transfer to a small saucepan. Bring marinade to a boil, and then remove from heat.

4. Place trout on the prepared grill. Baste fish with remaining marinade sauce while grilling. Cook approximately 5 minutes on each side, or until tender and easily flaked.

SANE   Free Tools: SANESolution.com/Tools   Superfoods: store.SANESolution.com

Asian Trout

Total Time: 20 min
Prep: 10 min
Cook: 10 min

8 Servings
2 Nutrient-Dense Protein Per Serving
1 Whole-Food Fat Per Serving

Ingredients

- 8 (6 ounce) fillets boneless, skinless rainbow trout
- 1 tablespoon and 1 teaspoon soy sauce
- salt and pepper to taste
- 2 teaspoons white sugar
- 2 teaspoons extra virgin coconut oil
- 2 teaspoons minced garlic
- 2 teaspoons minced fresh ginger
- 8 green onions, chopped

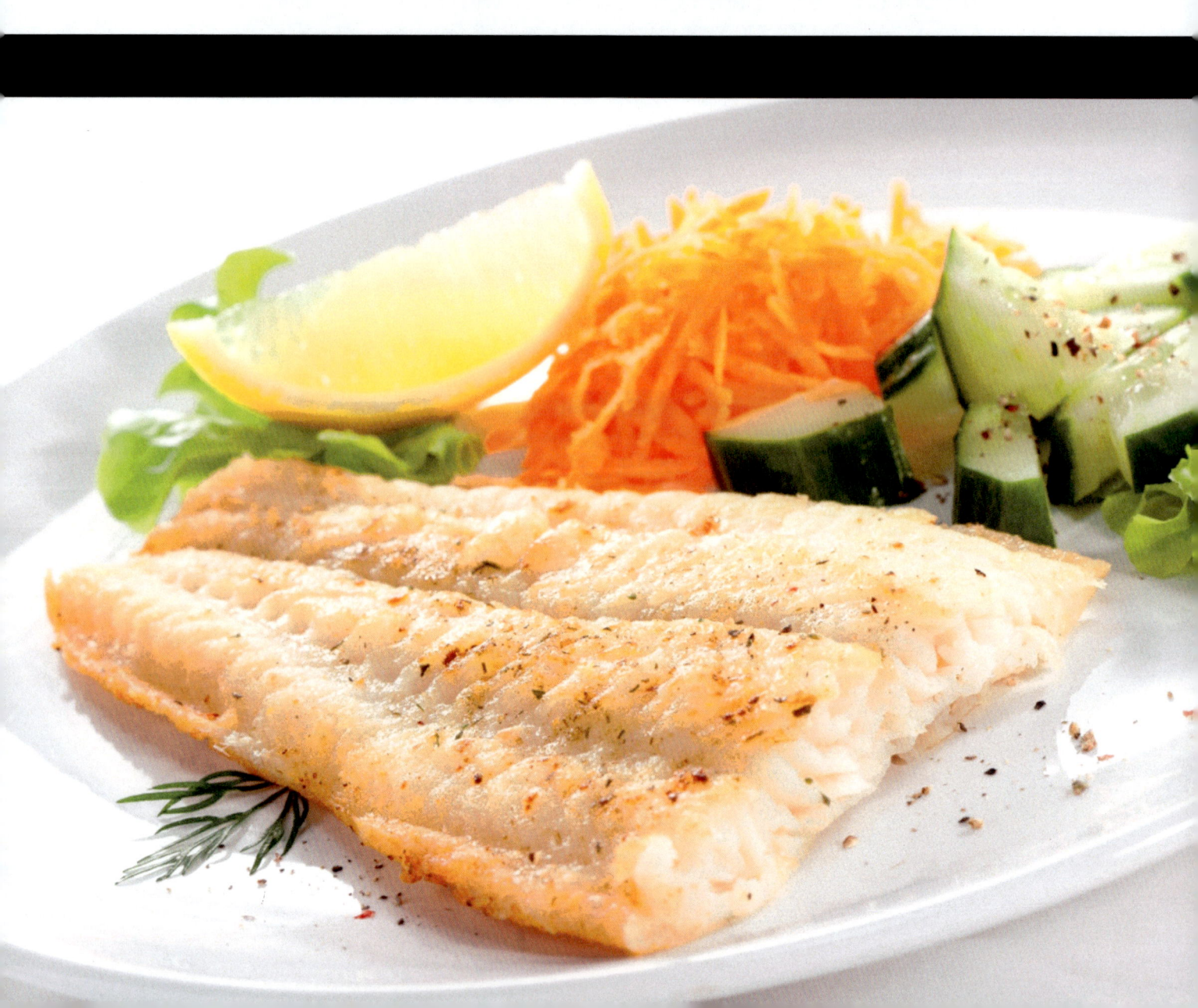

Directions

1. Rub trout fillets with soy sauce. Season with salt, pepper, and sugar; set aside.

2. Heat extra virgin coconut oil in a large skillet over medium-high heat. Add garlic, ginger, and green onions; cook and stir until golden brown. Add trout fillets and cook until browned and crispy, about 3 minutes. Turn fillets over, and continue cooking until the fish flakes easily with a fork, about 3 minutes more.

SANE Free Tools: SANESolution.com/Tools   Superfoods: store.SANESolution.com

Tuna

15-Minute Ahi

Total Time: 15 min
Prep: 10 min
Cook: 5 min

8 Servings
1 Nutrient-Dense Protein Per Serving
1 Whole-Food Fat Per Serving

Ingredients

- 2 pounds sashimi grade yellowfin tuna
- kosher salt to taste
- fresh ground black pepper to taste
- 1 cup Italian seasoned bread crumbs
- 1/4 cup and 2 tablespoons extra virgin coconut oil

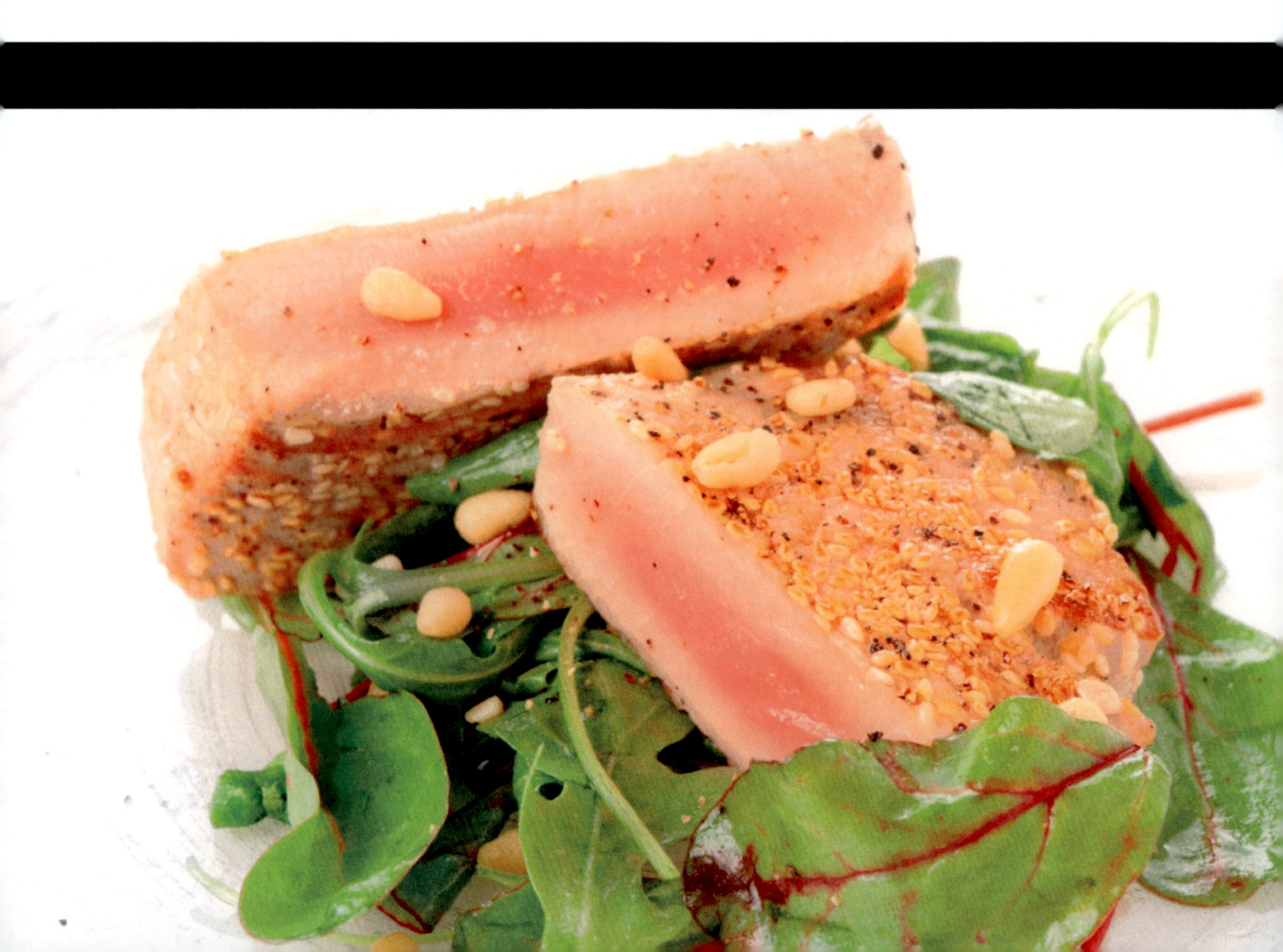

Directions

1. With a sharp knife, cut the tuna into 4 large pieces for appetizer portion, 2 large pieces for dinner portion. Use your judgment on what shape you want to cut your tuna because not all tuna is the same size or shape. However, the shape should somewhat resemble a miniature brick.

2. Season the tuna pieces with salt and pepper. Coat lightly on all sides with bread crumbs. Heat extra virgin coconut oil in a large heavy skillet over high heat. The pan should be as hot as you can get it. Place the tuna in the pan, and sear on each side for about 45 seconds for small portions, or 1 minute for large. Remove from pan. The tuna will be very rare.

3. Slice each 'brick' into 1/4 inch thick slices, and fan out on a serving plate. Enjoy plain, or with the condiments of your choice.

SANE   Free Tools: SANESolution.com/Tools   Superfoods: store.SANESolution.com

Horseradish Tuna

Total Time: 11 min
Prep: 5 min
Cook: 6 min

8 Servings
1 Nutrient-Dense Protein Per Serving
2 Whole-Food Fat Per Serving

Ingredients

- 8 (8 ounce) fresh tuna steaks
- 1 tablespoon and 1 teaspoon extra virgin coconut oil
- 1/2 cup soy sauce
- 1/2 cup seasoned rice vinegar
- 1/4 cup finely grated raw horseradish root, or more to taste
- 16 cherry tomatoes, sliced
- 2 teaspoons hot chile paste (such as sambal oelek)
- 1/4 cup minced green onion

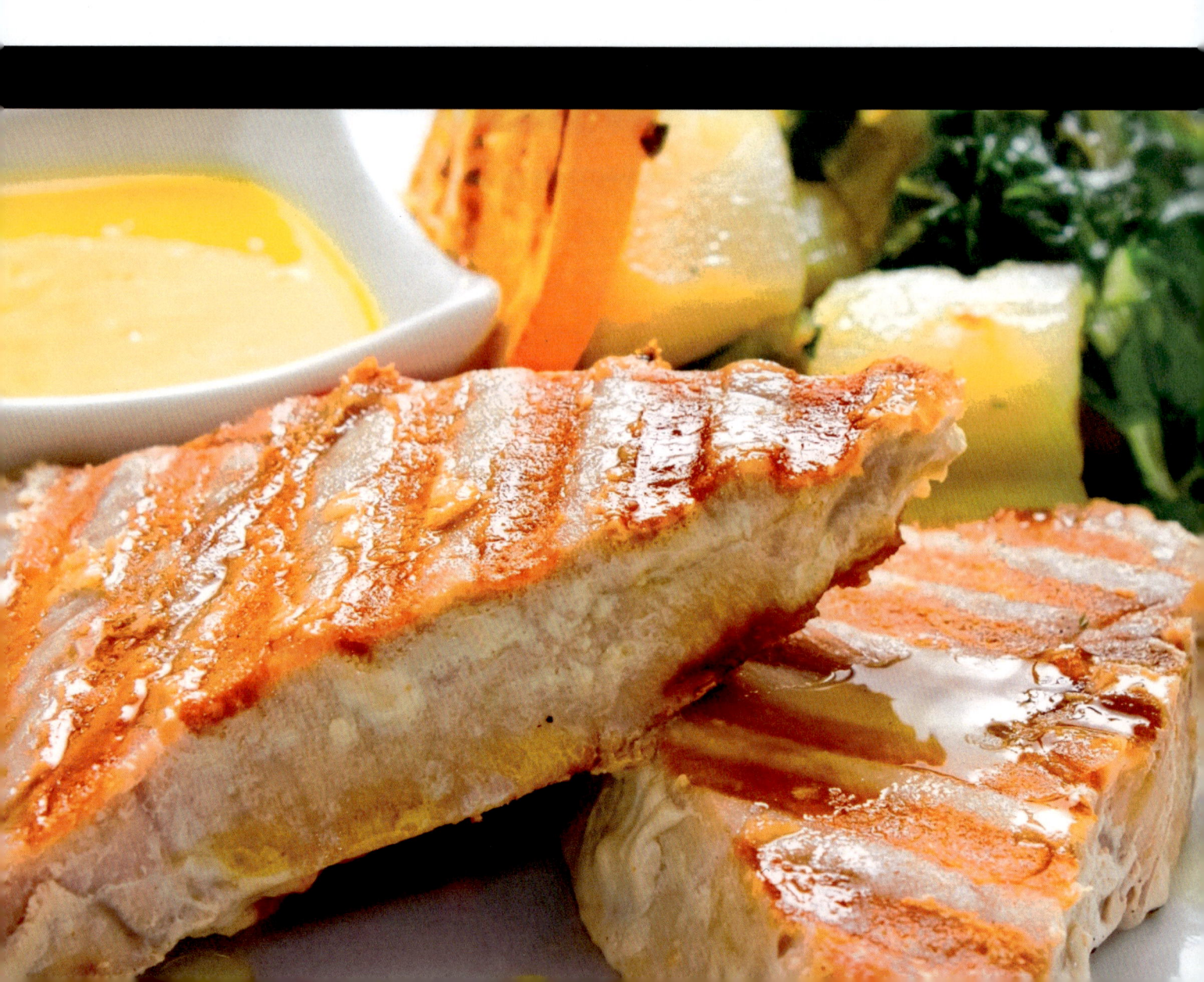

Directions

1. Preheat an outdoor grill for high heat, and lightly oil the grate. Lightly oil steaks with melted extra virgin coconut oil.

2. Stir soy sauce, rice vinegar, horseradish, cherry tomatoes, and hot chile paste in a bowl until well combined. Let sit for 20 minutes.

3. Place steaks over hottest part of the grill and cook for 3 minutes per side. Transfer to a plate. Spoon soy sauce mixture over steaks and garnish with green onion.

SANE   Free Tools: SANESolution.com/Tools   Superfoods: store.SANESolution.com

Blackened Tuna

Total Time: 20 min
Prep: 10 min
Cook: 10 min

8 Servings
1 Nutrient-Dense Protein Per Serving
2 Whole-Food Fat Per Serving

Ingredients

- 2 pounds fresh tuna steaks, 1 inch thick
- 2 tablespoons and 2 teaspoons Cajun seasoning
- 2 tablespoons and 2 teaspoons extra virgin coconut oil
- 2 tablespoons and 2 teaspoons butter

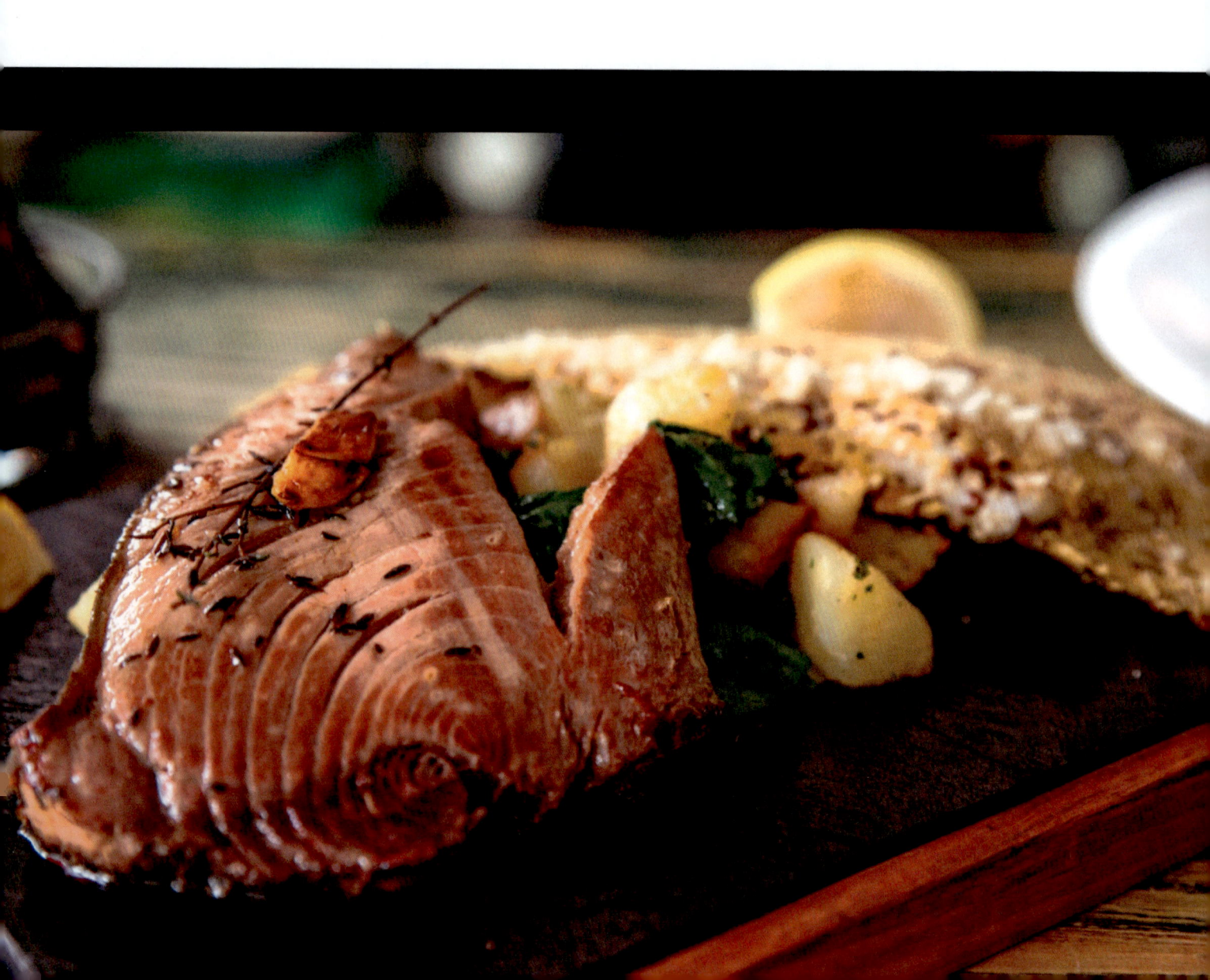

Directions

1. Generously coat tuna with Cajun seasoning.

2. Heat oil and butter in a large skillet over high heat. Right before oil starts smoking, place steaks in pan. Cook on one side for 3 to 4 minutes, or until blackened. Turn steaks, and cook for 3 to 4 minutes, or to desired doneness.

SANE   Free Tools: SANESolution.com/Tools   Superfoods: store.SANESolution.com

Succulent Tuna Steaks

Total Time: 21 min
Prep: 10 min
Cook: 11 min

8 Servings
1 Nutrient-Dense Protein Per Serving
1 Whole-Food Fat Per Serving

Ingredients

- 1/2 cup orange juice
- 1/2 cup soy sauce
- 1/4 cup extra virgin coconut oil
- 2 tablespoons lemon juice
- 1/4 cup chopped fresh parsley
- 2 cloves garlic, minced
- 1 teaspoon chopped fresh oregano
- 1 teaspoon ground black pepper
- 8 (4 ounce) tuna steaks

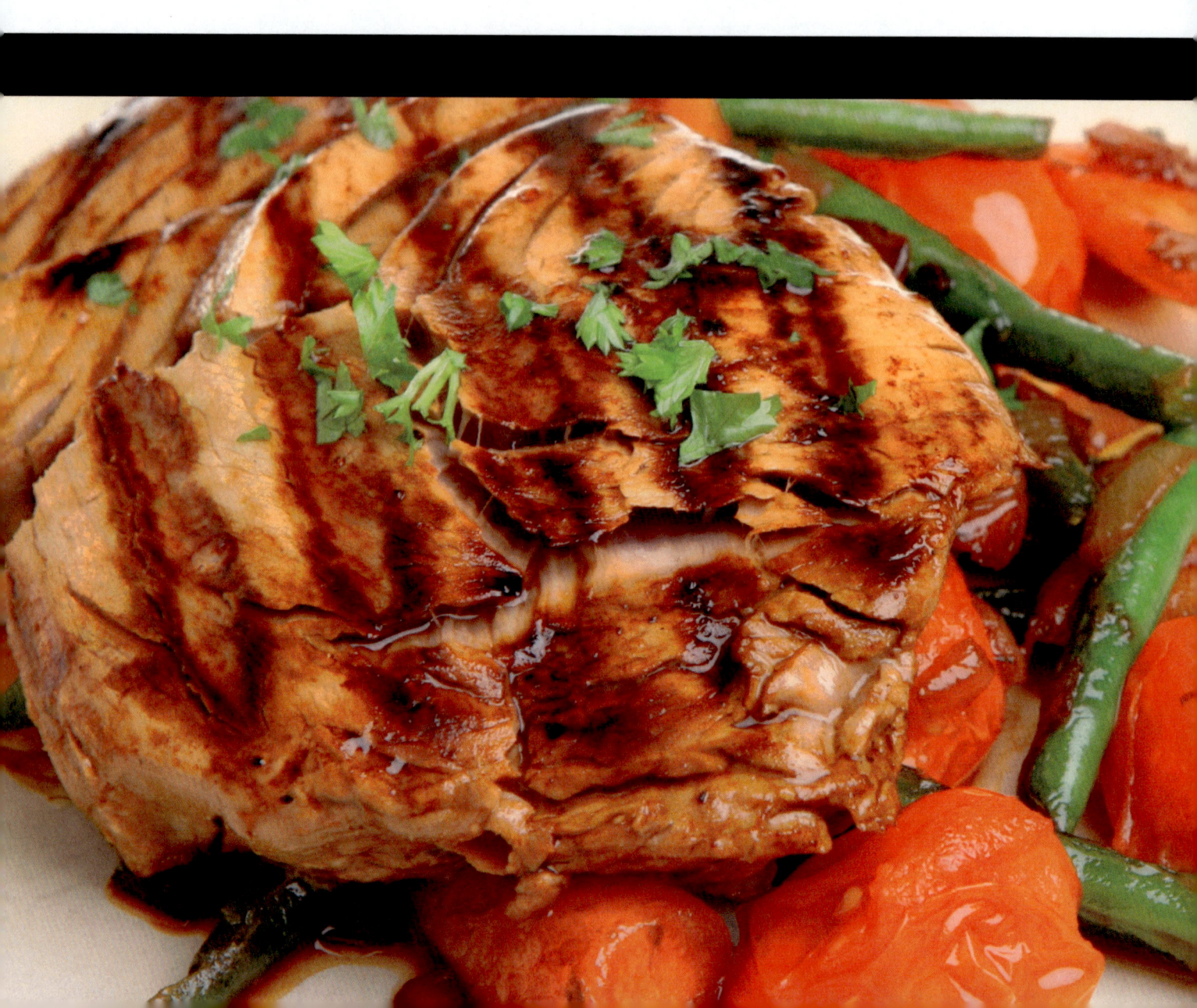

Directions

1. In a large non-reactive dish, mix together the orange juice, soy sauce, coconut oil, lemon juice, parsley, garlic, oregano, and pepper. Place the tuna steaks in the marinade and turn to coat. Cover, and refrigerate for at least 30 minutes.

2. Preheat grill for high heat.

3. Lightly oil grill grate. Cook the tuna steaks for 5 to 6 minutes, then turn and baste with the marinade. Cook for an additional 5 minutes, or to desired doneness. Discard any remaining marinade.

SANE   Free Tools: SANESolution.com/Tools   Superfoods: store.SANESolution.com

Poached Tuna Steaks

Total Time: 30 min
Prep: 15 min
Cook: 15 min

8 Servings
1 Nutrient-Dense Protein Per Serving
1 Whole-Food Fat Per Serving

Ingredients

- 6 cups water
- 1/4 cup fresh lemon juice
- 1 tablespoon and 1 teaspoon cayenne pepper
- salt and pepper to taste
- 8 (4 ounce) albacore tuna steaks
- 12 kumquats – rinsed, seeded and sliced
- 1-1/3 cups chopped fresh cilantro

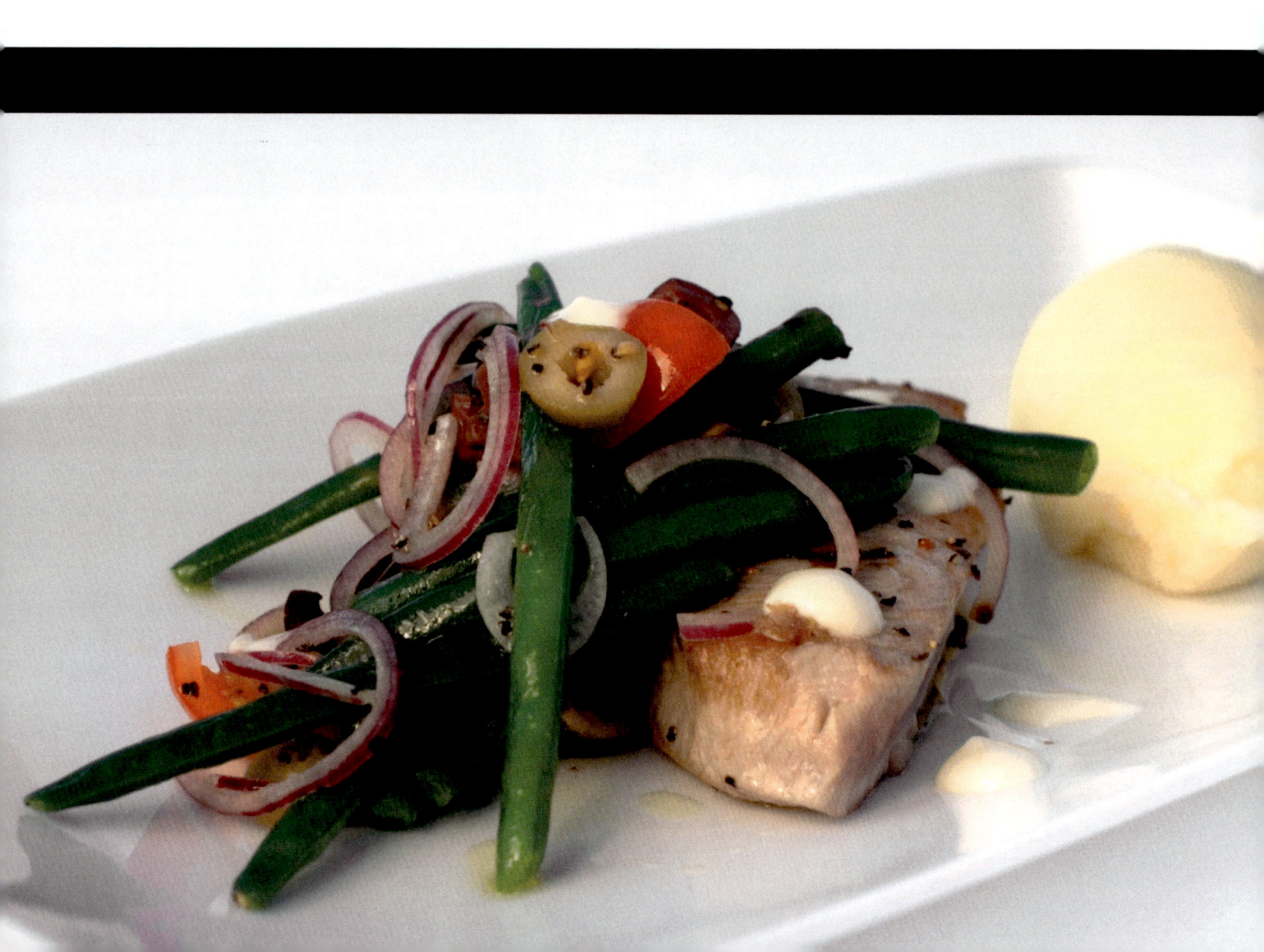

Directions

1. In a medium saucepan over medium heat, mix water, lemon juice, and cayenne pepper. Season with salt and pepper. Bring to a gentle boil.

2. Place tuna steaks into the mixture, and sprinkle with kumquats and cilantro. Cook 15 minutes, until fish is easily flaked with a fork.

SANE   Free Tools: SANESolution.com/Tools   Superfoods: store.SANESolution.com

Quick Tuna Steaks

Total Time: 11 min
Prep: 5 min
Cook: 6 min

8 Servings
2 Nutrient-Dense Protein Per Serving
1 Whole-Food Fat Per Serving

Ingredients

- 1/3 cup extra virgin coconut oil
- 1/4 cup grated lemon zest
- 1 tablespoon and 1 teaspoon ground coriander
- 2-1/2 teaspoons ground black pepper
- 1 tablespoon ground ginger
- 2 teaspoons salt
- 1 teaspoon ground cinnamon
- 8 (5 ounce) tuna steaks, about 1 inch thick

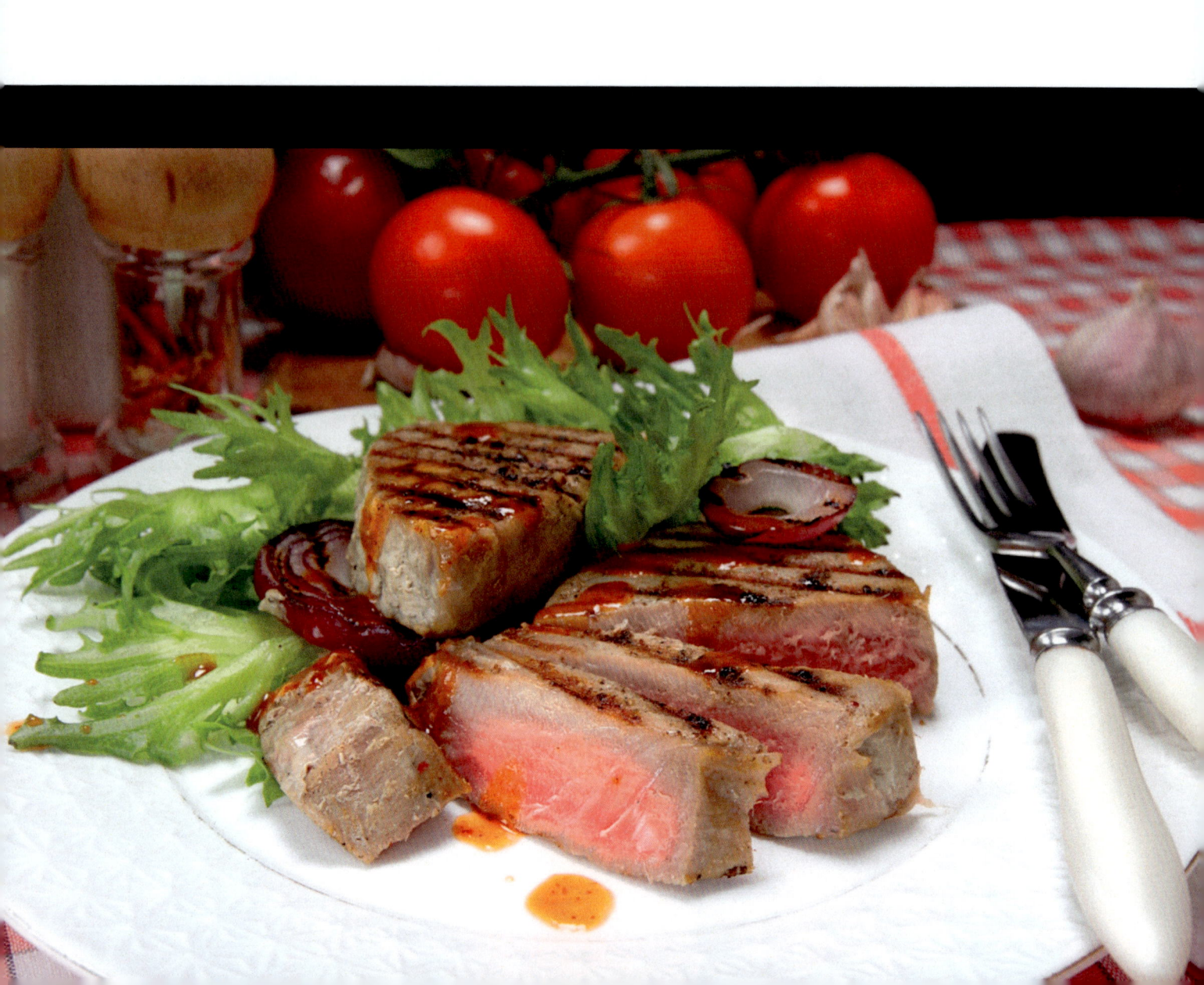

Directions

1. Whisk 2 tablespoons melted extra virgin coconut oil, lemon zest, coriander, black pepper, ginger, salt, and cinnamon in a small bowl; rub tuna steaks with spice mixture.

2. Heat 1 tablespoon extra virgin coconut oil in a large skillet over medium-high heat. Sear tuna in the hot oil until browned but still pink in the center, about 3 minutes on each side.

SANE Free Tools: SANESolution.com/Tools   Superfoods: store.SANESolution.com

Tuna Citrus

Total Time: 20 min
Prep: 10 min
Cook: 10 min

8 Servings
2 Nutrient-Dense Protein Per Serving
1 Whole-Food Fat Per Serving

Ingredients

- 2 cups orange juice
- 2 tablespoons extra virgin coconut oil
- 1 tablespoon and 1 teaspoon oregano, dried
- 1 tablespoon and 1 teaspoon finely chopped fresh parsley
- salt and ground black pepper to taste
- 8 (6 ounce) fresh tuna steaks

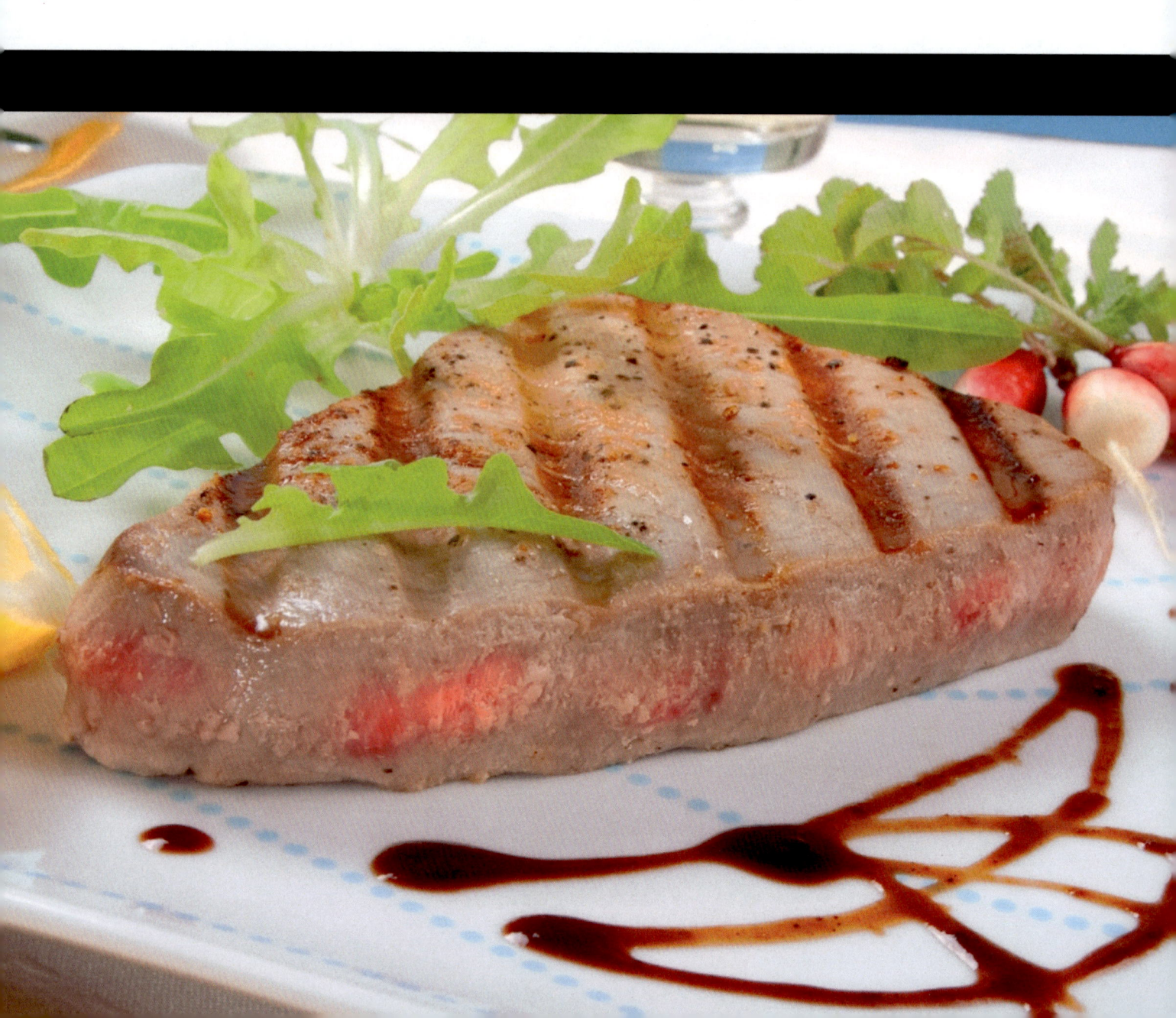

Directions

1. In a large bowl, combine orange juice, extra virgin coconut oil, oregano, parsley, salt, and pepper. Mix well. Place the tuna steaks in the bowl, turn to coat both sides with marinade; cover and refrigerate 30 minutes.

2. Preheat an outdoor grill for medium-high heat.

3. Remove tuna from the marinade and shake off excess. Place tuna onto preheated grill and cook to desired doneness, about 5 minutes per inch for medium-rare or 10 minutes per inch for medium-well.

SANE   Free Tools: SANESolution.com/Tools   Superfoods: store.SANESolution.com

Tuna Tarragon

Total Time: 20 min
Prep: 5 min
Cook: 15 min

8 Servings
2 Nutrient-Dense Protein Per Serving
3 Whole-Food Fat Per Serving

Ingredients

- 1/4 cup and 2 tablespoons extra virgin coconut oil
- 4 cloves garlic, peeled and minced
- 1/4 cup tarragon vinegar
- 1 teaspoon dried tarragon
- freshly ground black pepper to taste
- 3 pounds fresh tuna steaks

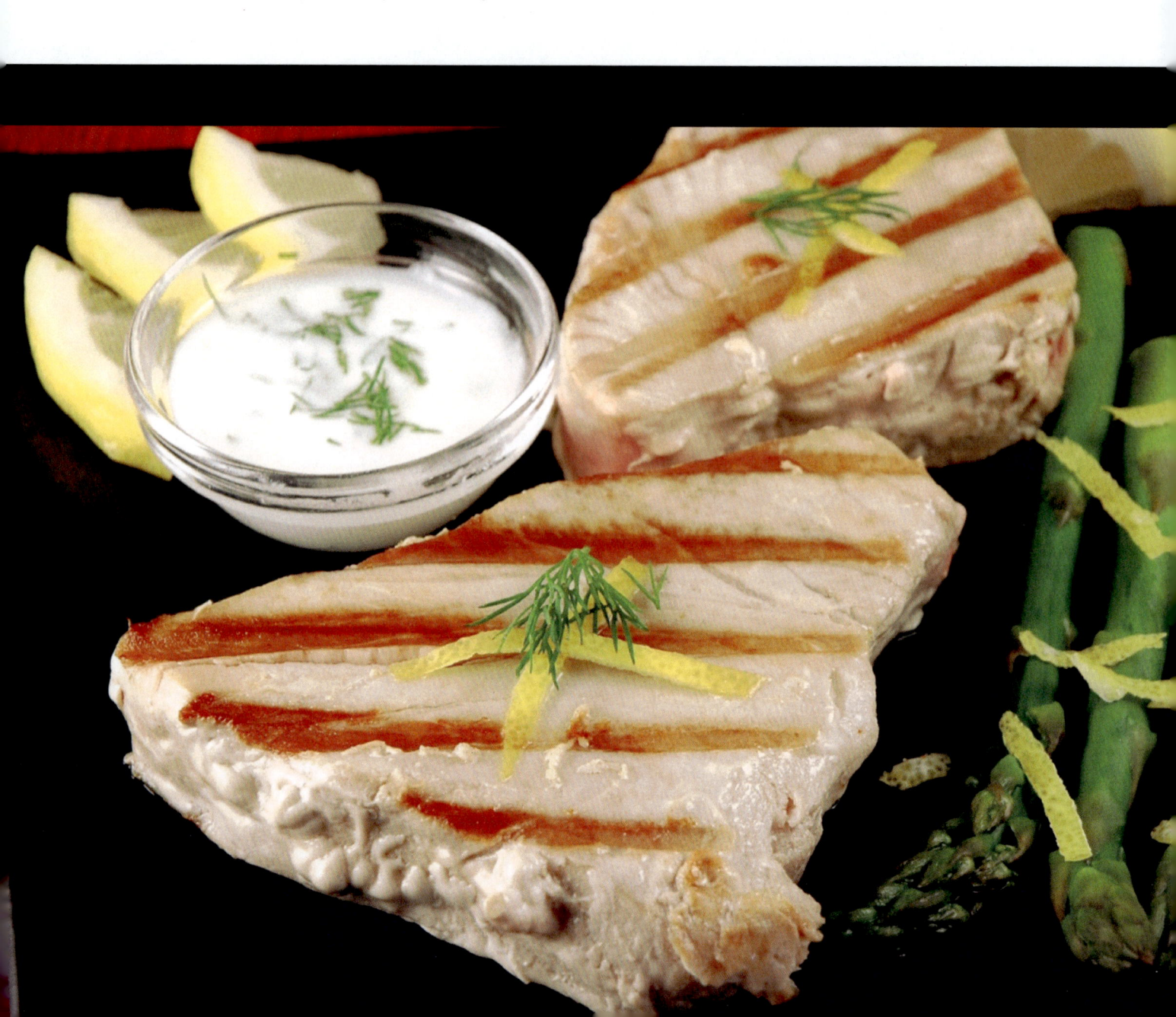

Directions

1. In a medium bowl, whisk together extra virgin coconut oil, garlic, tarragon vinegar, dried tarragon and pepper. Place tuna steaks into the mixture. Cover and marinate in the refrigerator at least 4 hours.

2. Preheat an outdoor grill for high heat and lightly oil grate.

3. Grill tuna steaks 8 to 10 minutes per side, until the tuna flakes easily and is opaque in the center.

SANE   Free Tools: SANESolution.com/Tools   Superfoods: store.SANESolution.com

Wasabi Tuna

Total Time: 10 min
Prep: 5 min
Cook: 5 min

8 Servings
2 Nutrient-Dense Protein Per Serving
1 Whole-Food Fat Per Serving

Ingredients

- 1/4 cup all-natural reduced-fat mayonnaise
- 1 tablespoon wasabi paste
- 2 teaspoons Chinese five-spice powder
- 2 tablespoons low-sodium soy sauce
- 8 (6 ounce) yellowfin tuna fillets
- 2 tablespoons rice vinegar
- 2 tablespoons low-sodium soy sauce
- 1/4 cup toasted sesame seeds

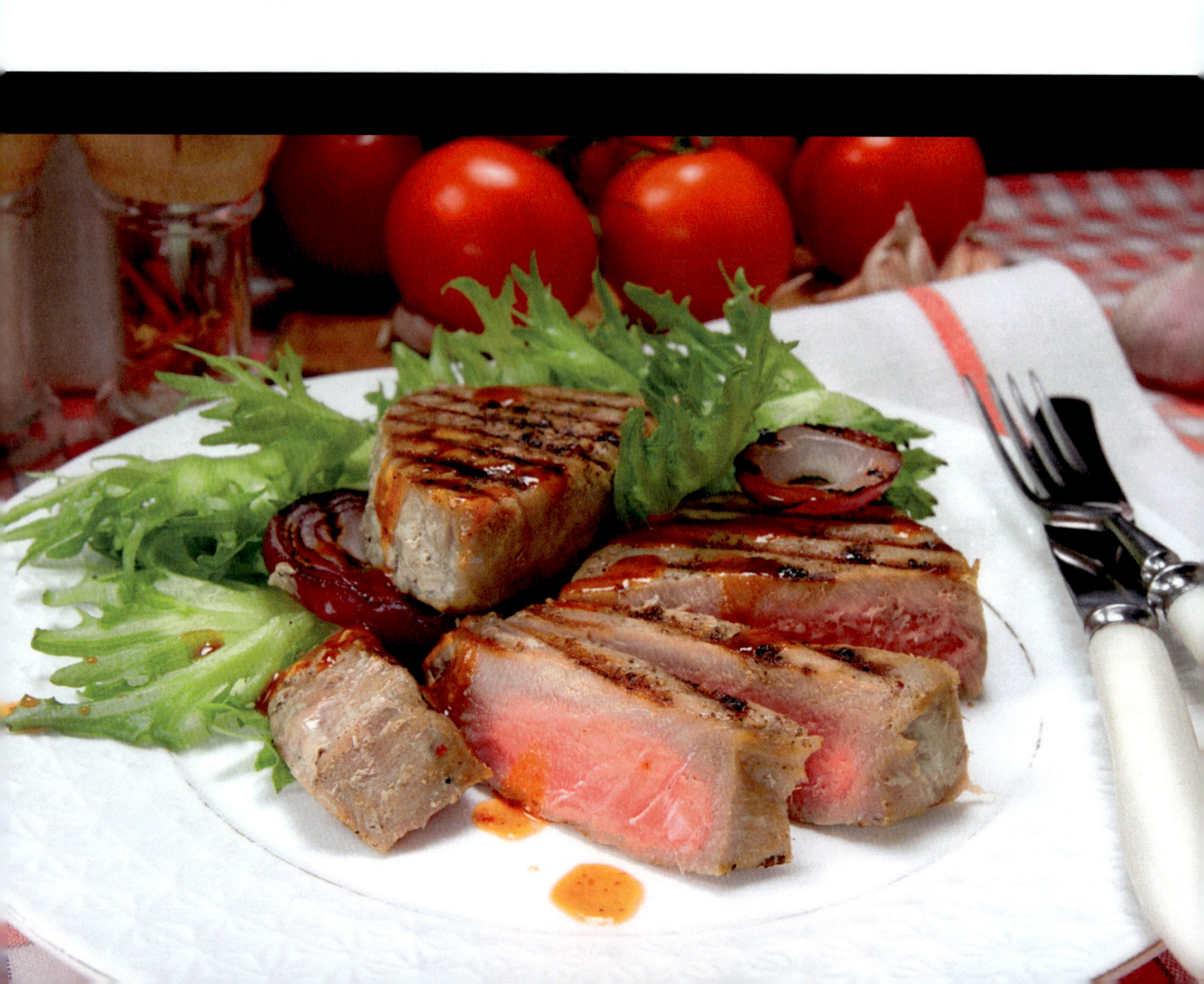

Directions

1. Mix together the mayonnaise, wasabi paste, five-spice powder, and 1 tablespoon soy sauce in a small bowl.

2. Lay the tuna fillets into a glass baking dish. Pour the rice vinegar and 1 tablespoon soy sauce over the tuna. Spread the mayonnaise mixture evenly over both sides of each piece of fish. Cover the dish and refrigerate 15 to 30 minutes.

3. Prepare a skillet with cooking spray and place over medium-high heat. Sprinkle the sesame seeds evenly over both sides of the fillets. Lay the tuna gently into the skillet. Grill to desired level of doneness, about 2 minutes per side for medium-rare. Serve immediately.

Other Fish & Seafood

Butter Herb Catfish

Total Time: 30 min
Prep: 10 min
Cook: 20 min

8 Servings
1 Nutrient-Dense Protein Per Serving
1 Whole-Food Fat Per Serving

Ingredients

- 8 (6 ounce) catfish fillets
- 1/4 cup dried parsley
- 1-1/2 teaspoons paprika
- 1 teaspoon dried thyme
- 1 teaspoon dried oregano
- 1 teaspoon dried basil
- 1 teaspoon ground black pepper
- 1/4 cup lemon juice
- 2 tablespoons butter, melted
- 1/2 teaspoon garlic powder

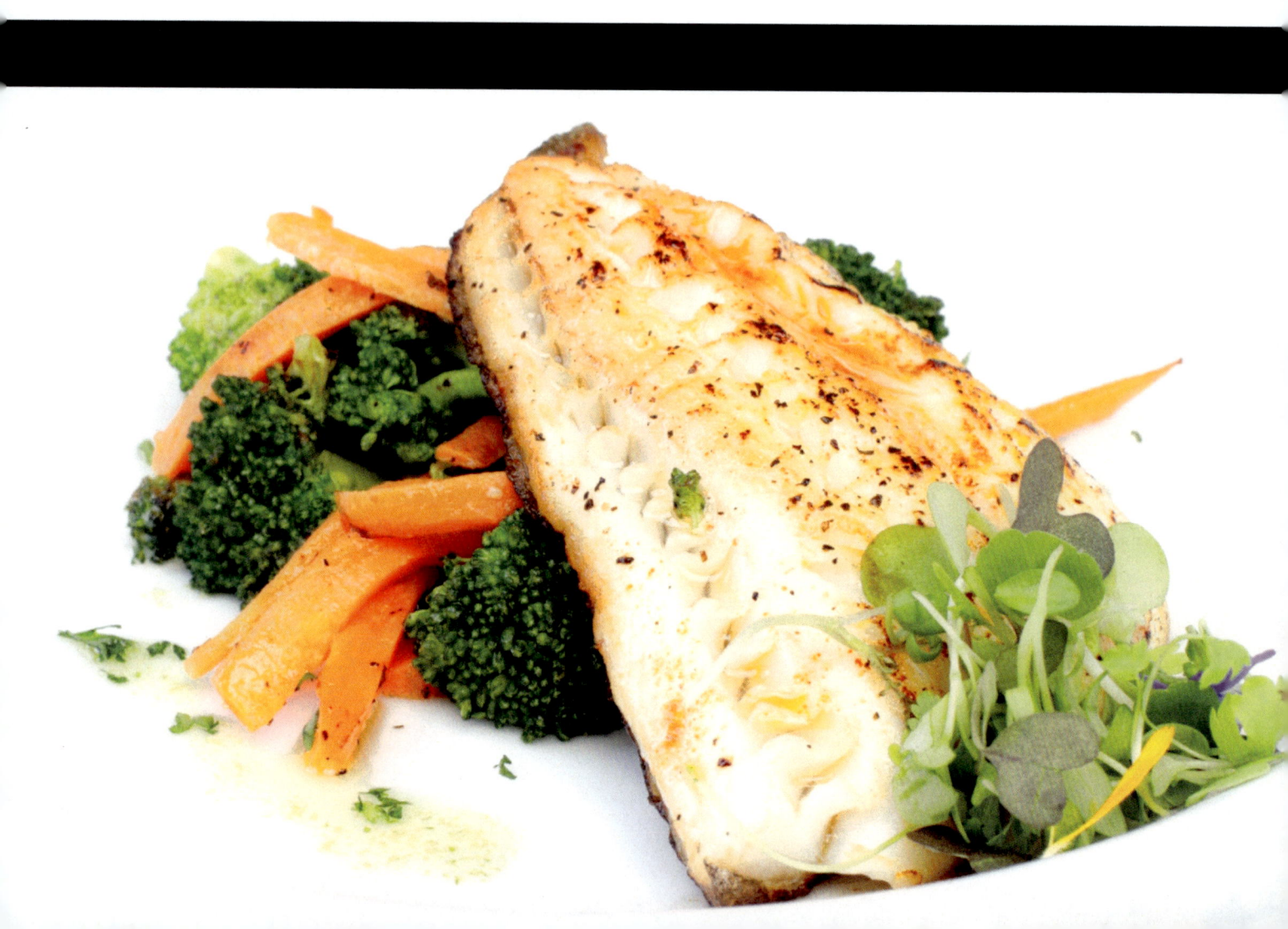

Directions

1. Preheat oven to 350 degrees F (175 degrees C).

2. Arrange catfish fillets in a 9×13-inch baking dish. Combine parsley, paprika, thyme, oregano, basil, and black pepper in a small bowl; sprinkle herb mixture over fish. Mix lemon juice, butter, and garlic powder in another bowl; drizzle butter mixture over fish.

3. Bake in preheated oven until fish is easily flaked with a fork, about 20 minutes.

SANE — Free Tools: SANESolution.com/Tools — Superfoods: store.SANESolution.com

Venetian Catfish

Total Time: 40 min
Prep: 20 min
Cook: 20 min

8 Servings
1 Nutrient-Dense Protein Per Serving
2 Whole-Food Fat Per Serving

Ingredients

- 1/4 cup extra virgin coconut oil
- 5/8 onion, diced
- 5/8 green bell pepper, diced
- 1-1/4 carrot, peeled and diced
- 10-1/2 (4 ounce) fillets catfish fillets
- salt and black pepper to taste
- 1-1/4 teaspoons Italian seasoning
- garlic powder to taste
- 1-1/4 (14.4 ounce) cans diced Italian tomatoes
- 1-1/4 (8 ounce) cans tomato sauce
- 2/3 cup dry white wine

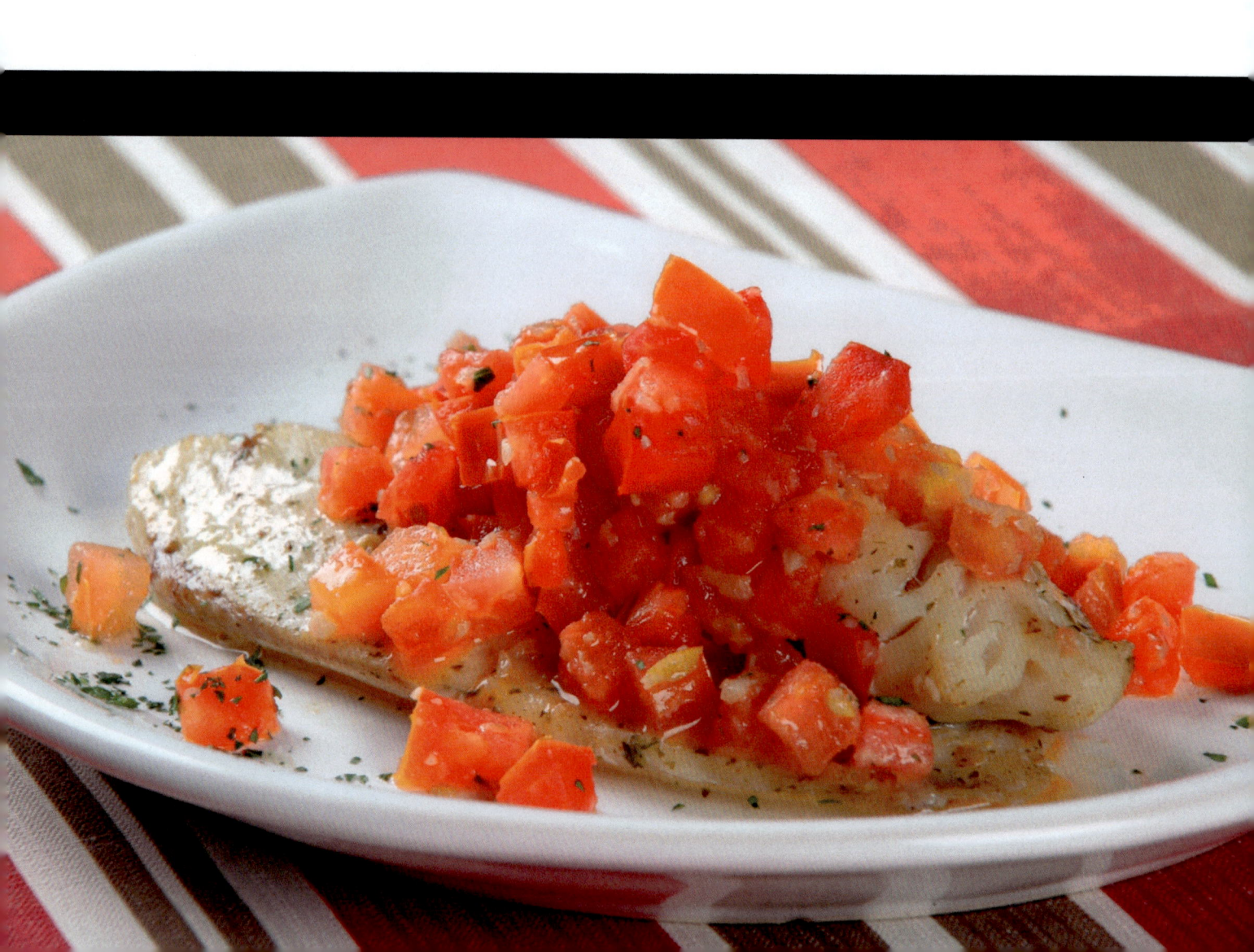

Directions

1. Place 1 tablespoon of oil in a heavy bottomed skillet over medium heat. Saute onion, green pepper, and carrot until golden brown; remove from the pan. Using the remaining 2 tablespoons of oil, sear all of the fillets on both sides. Lay all of the fillets into the skillet, sprinkle with salt, pepper, Italian seasoning, and garlic powder. Top with the sautéed vegetables, and pour on the diced tomatoes, tomato sauce, and white wine.

2. Bring to a simmer, and cook gently until the sauce has thickened slightly, and fish flakes easily with a fork, about 10 minutes.

SANE Free Tools: SANESolution.com/Tools   Superfoods: store.SANESolution.com

Greek Catfish

Total Time: 35 min
Prep: 15 min
Cook: 20 min

8 Servings
2 Nutrient-Dense Protein Per Serving
2 Whole-Food Fat Per Serving

Ingredients

- 8 (8 ounce) fillets catfish
- Greek seasoning, or to taste
- 5 ounces crumbled feta cheese
- 6 toothpicks
- 1 tablespoon and 1 teaspoon dried mint
- 2 tablespoons and 2 teaspoons extra virgin coconut oil

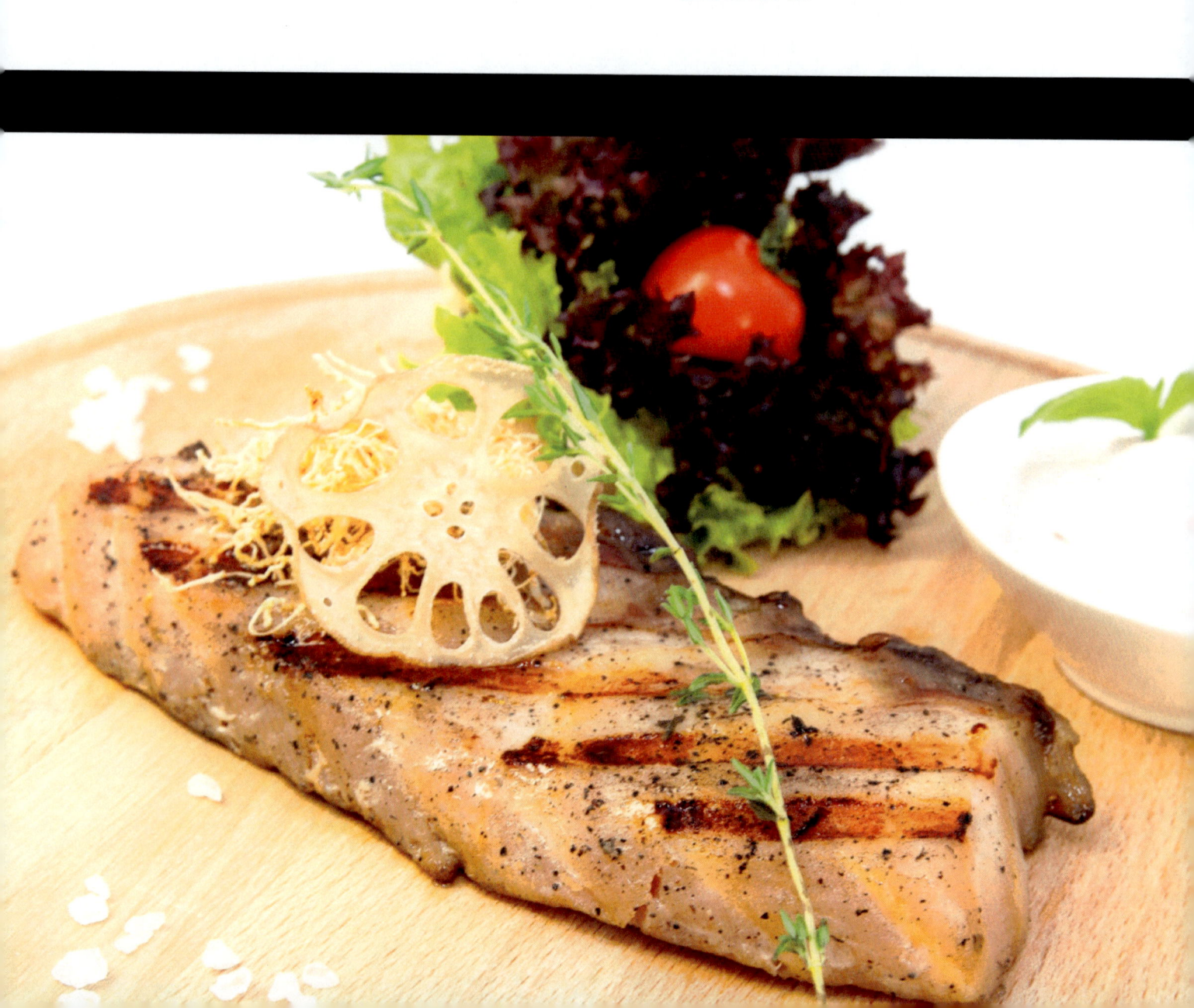

Directions

1. Preheat grill for medium heat and lightly oil the grate.

2. Season both sides of each catfish fillet with Greek seasoning. Sprinkle feta cheese and mint over one side of each fillet; drizzle olive oil over the cheese and mint. Beginning with narrower end, roll fish tightly around the filling and secure with a toothpick.

3. Cook on preheated grill until the fish flakes easily with a fork, 20 to 25 minutes.

Crab Encrusted Grouper

Total Time: 40 min
Prep: 10 min
Cook: 30 min

8 Servings
2 Nutrient-Dense Protein Per Serving
1 Whole-Food Fat Per Serving

Ingredients

- 1/4 cup Parmesan cheese flavored bread crumbs
- 1/4 cup chopped red bell pepper
- 1/4 cup chopped yellow bell pepper
- 4 green onions, chopped
- 1/2 jalapeno pepper, seeded and minced
- 1/2 cup butter, melted
- 2 (6 ounce) cans crabmeat, drained and flaked
- 1/4 cup shredded mozzarella cheese
- 8 (6 ounce) fillets grouper

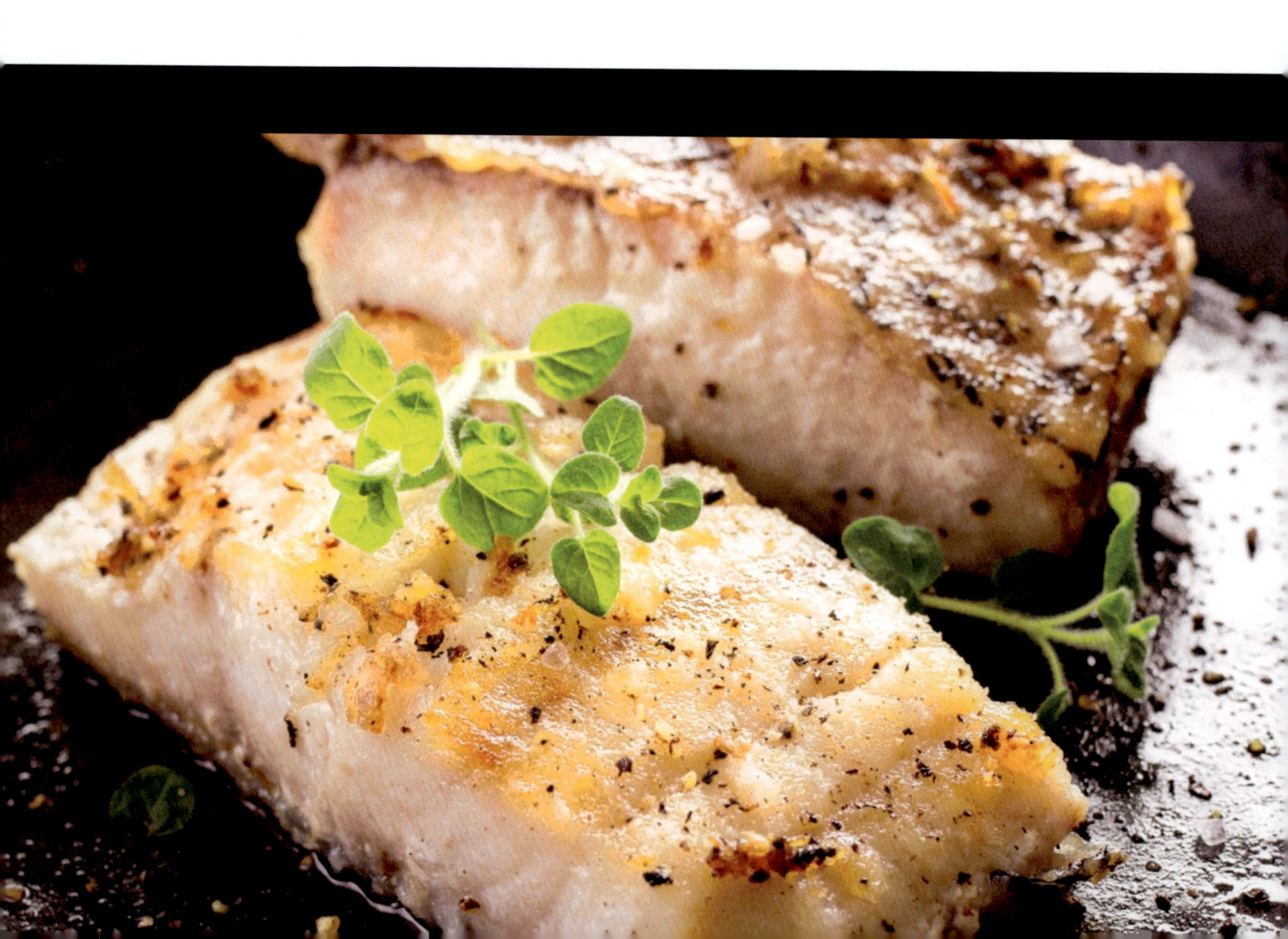

Directions

1. Preheat the oven to 375 degrees F (190 degrees C).

2. In a medium bowl, stir together the bread crumbs, red pepper, yellow pepper, green onions, jalapeno, butter, crabmeat, and mozzarella cheese. Arrange grouper fillets in a single layer in a 9×13 inch baking dish. Spread the crumb topping evenly over the fish.

3. Bake for 30 minutes in the preheated oven, or until fish is easily flaked with a fork. If you have thin fillets, you may broil for 10 minutes instead of baking.

SANE   Free Tools: SANESolution.com/Tools   Superfoods: store.SANESolution.com

Quick Barbecued Sea Bass

Total Time: 20 min
Prep: 5 min
Cook: 15 min

8 Servings
2 Nutrient-Dense Protein Per Serving
1 Whole-Food Fat Per Serving

Ingredients

- 1/4 cup lemon juice
- 1 tablespoon and 1 teaspoon extra virgin coconut oil
- salt and pepper to taste
- 4 bay leaf
- 4 pounds fresh sea bass

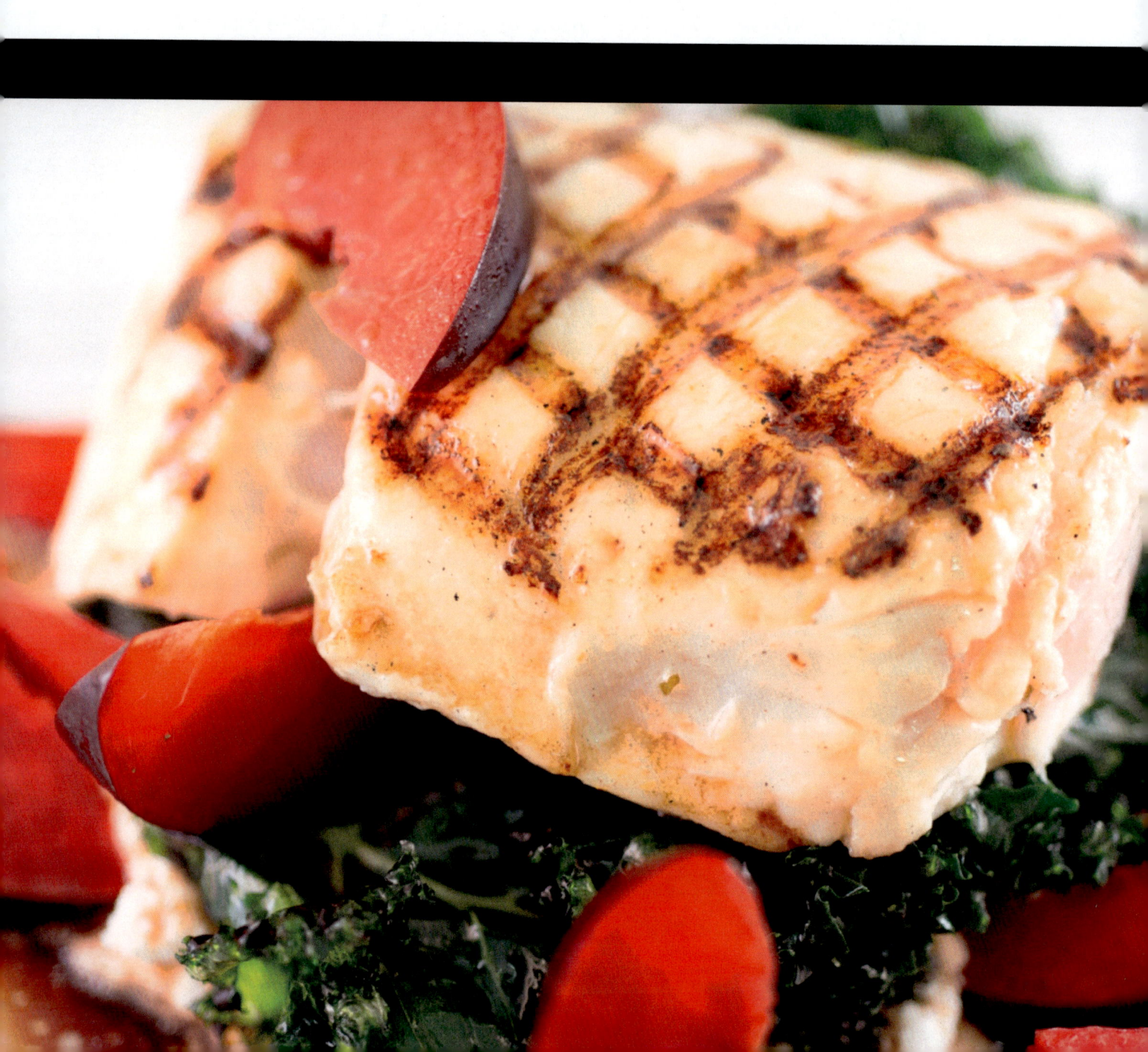

Directions

1. Preheat an outdoor grill for medium heat and lightly oil grate.

2. In a small bowl, stir together lemon juice, extra virgin coconut oil, salt, pepper and bay leaf. Rub fish with mixture inside and out.

3. Grill the fish over medium heat for 8 to 10 minutes, flipping halfway through. Fish is done when it flakes easily with a fork.

SANE Free Tools: SANESolution.com/Tools   Superfoods: store.SANESolution.com

Baked Basil Halibut

Total Time: 30 min
Prep: 15 min
Cook: 15 min

8 Servings
1 Nutrient-Dense Protein Per Serving
2 Whole-Food Fat Per Serving

Ingredients

- 1 tablespoon and 1 teaspoon extra virgin coconut oil
- 1-1/4 small onion, halved and thinly sliced
- 5/8 bell pepper, sliced thinly
- 11 ounces sliced fresh mushrooms
- 1-1/4 cloves chopped fresh garlic
- 2-3/4 medium zucchini, julienned
- 8 (6 ounce) halibut steaks
- 3/4 teaspoon dried basil
- 3/4 teaspoon salt, or to taste
- 3/4 teaspoon ground black pepper
- 1-1/4 medium tomato, thinly sliced

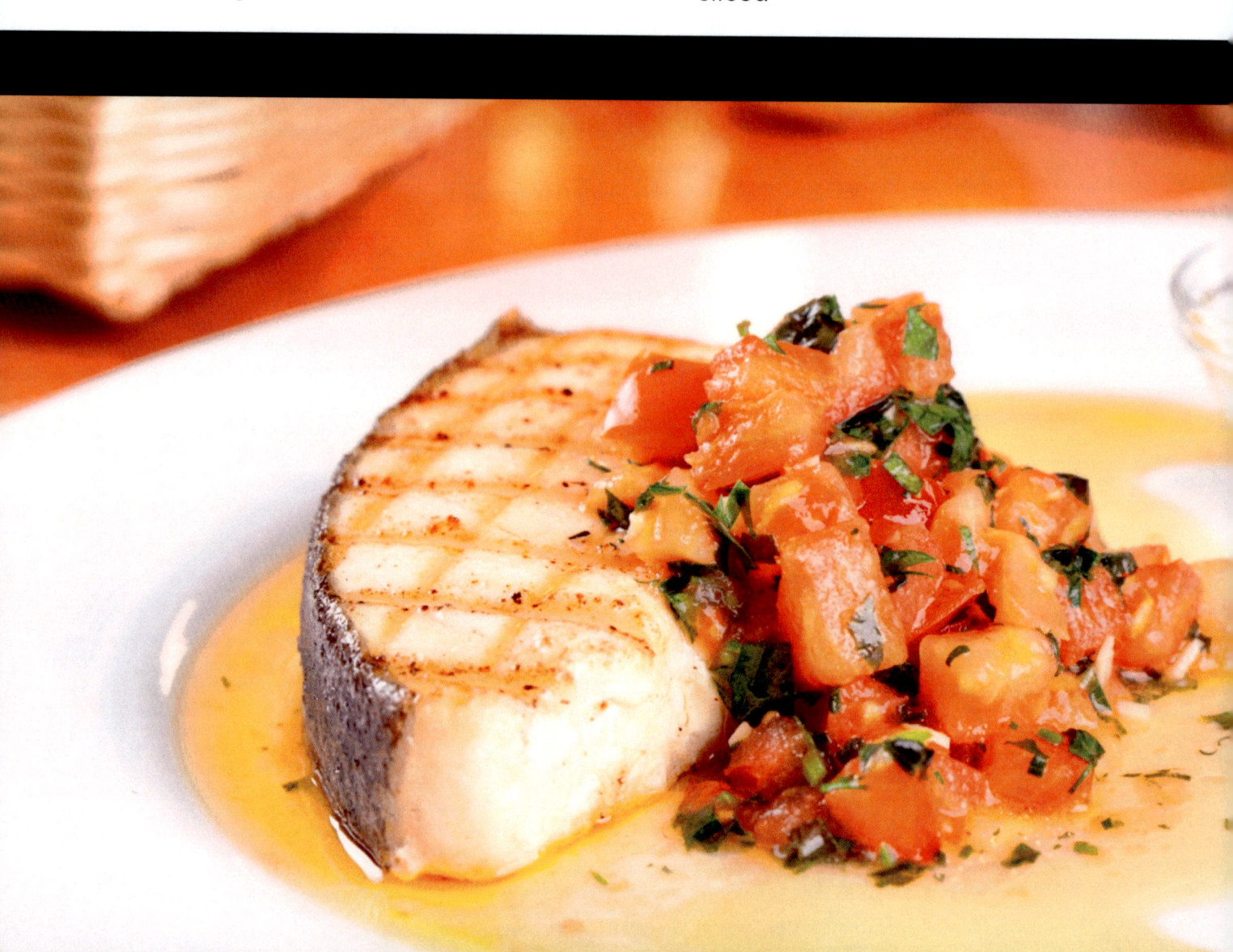

Directions

1. Preheat the oven to 400 degrees F (200 degrees C).

2. Heat the extra virgin coconut oil in a skillet over medium heat. Add the onion, bell pepper, mushrooms, garlic and zucchini. Cover, and cook stirring occasionally, until the onions are translucent, about 5 minutes.

3. Place halibut steaks into a shallow baking dish, and top with the sautéed vegetables. Season with basil, salt and pepper.

4. Bake for 10 minutes in the preheated oven, then remove the dish, and cover the fillets with a layer of sliced tomato. Return to the oven, and bake for an additional 10 minutes, or until fish flakes easily with a fork.

BBQ Halibut

Total Time: 25 min
Prep: 10 min
Cook: 15 min

8 Servings
2 Nutrient-Dense Protein Per Serving
1 Whole-Food Fat Per Serving

Ingredients

- 1/3 cup butter
- 1/3 cup brown sugar
- 5-1/4 cloves garlic, minced
- 2 tablespoons and 2 teaspoons lemon juice
- 1 tablespoon and 2-1/4 teaspoons soy sauce
- 1-1/4 teaspoons ground black pepper
- 2-3/4 (1 pound) halibut steak

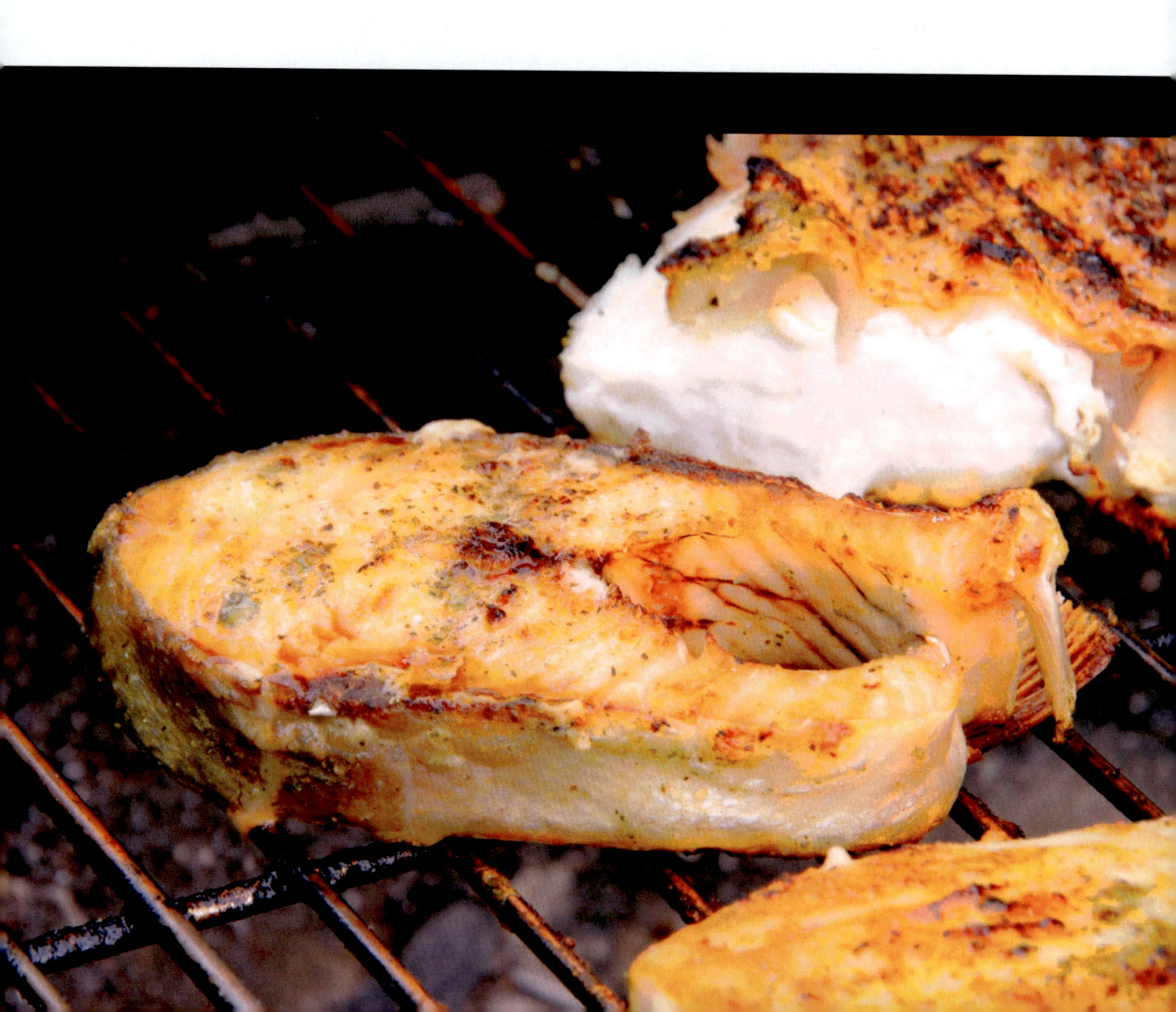

Directions

1. Preheat grill for medium-high heat.

2. Place butter, brown sugar, garlic, lemon juice, soy sauce, and pepper in a small saucepan. Warm over medium heat, stirring occasionally, until sugar is completely dissolved.

3. Lightly oil grill grate. Brush fish with brown sugar sauce, and place on grill. Cook for 5 minutes per side, or until fish can be easily flaked with a fork, basting with sauce. Discard remaining basting sauce.

SANE Free Tools: SANESolution.com/Tools   Superfoods: store.SANEsolution.com

Ginger Halibut

Total Time: 25 min
Prep: 15 min
Cook: 10 min

8 Servings
2 Nutrient-Dense Protein Per Serving
2 Whole-Food Fat Per Serving

Ingredients

- 4 pounds halibut fillet
- 1 tablespoon and 1 teaspoon coarse sea salt or kosher salt
- 1/4 cup minced fresh ginger
- 3/4 cup thinly sliced green onion
- 1/4 cup dark soy sauce
- 1/4 cup light soy sauce
- 1/2 cup extra virgin coconut oil
- 1 cup lightly packed fresh cilantro sprigs

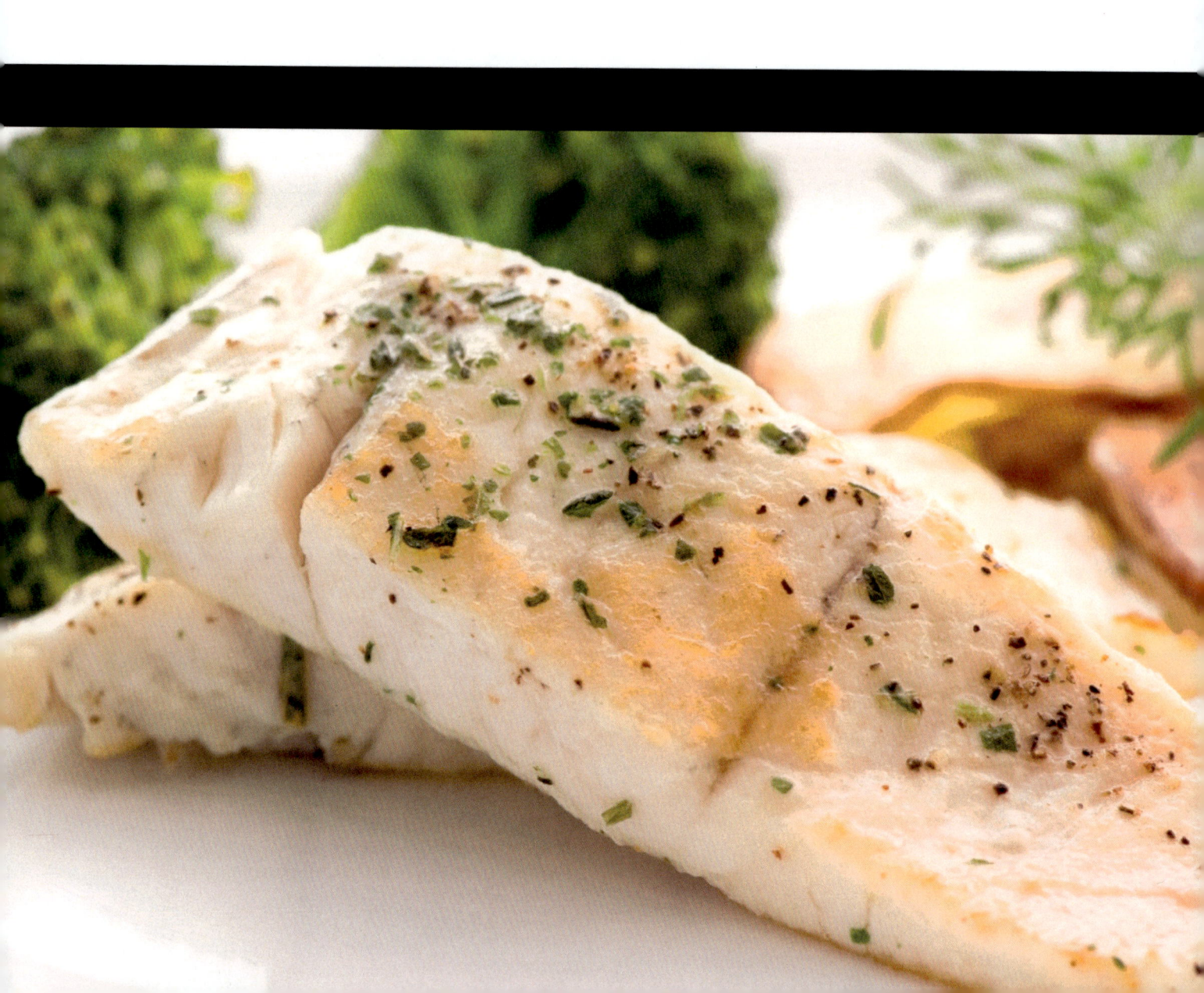

Directions

1. Pat halibut dry with paper towels. Rub both sides of fillet with salt. Scatter the ginger over the top of the fish and place onto a heatproof ceramic dish.

2. Place into a bamboo steamer set over several inches of gently boiling water, and cover. Gently steam for 10 to 12 minutes.

3. Pour accumulated water out of the dish and sprinkle the fillet with green onion. Drizzle both soy sauces over the surface of the fish.

4. Heat extra virgin coconut oil in a small skillet over medium-high heat until it starts to bubble. When the oil is hot, VERY carefully pour on top of the halibut fillet. The very hot oil will cause the green onions and water on top of the fish to pop and spatter all over; be VERY careful. Garnish with cilantro sprigs and serve immediately.

Pepper and Pesto Mahi Mahi

Total Time: 40 min
Prep: 20 min
Cook: 20 min

8 Servings
2 Nutrient-Dense Protein Per Serving
1 Whole-Food Fat Per Serving

Ingredients

- 1 cup white wine
- 2 shallot, minced
- 1/4 cup shredded Parmesan cheese
- 4 cloves garlic
- 2/3 cup chopped walnuts
- 2 tablespoons extra virgin coconut oil
- 1/2 cup packed fresh cilantro leaves
- 1/4 teaspoon ground black pepper
- 2 (12 ounce) jars roasted red bell peppers, drained
- 8 (6 ounce) mahi mahi fillets
- salt and ground black pepper to taste
- 2 tablespoons butter
- 1/4 teaspoon ground black pepper
- 1/2 teaspoon salt

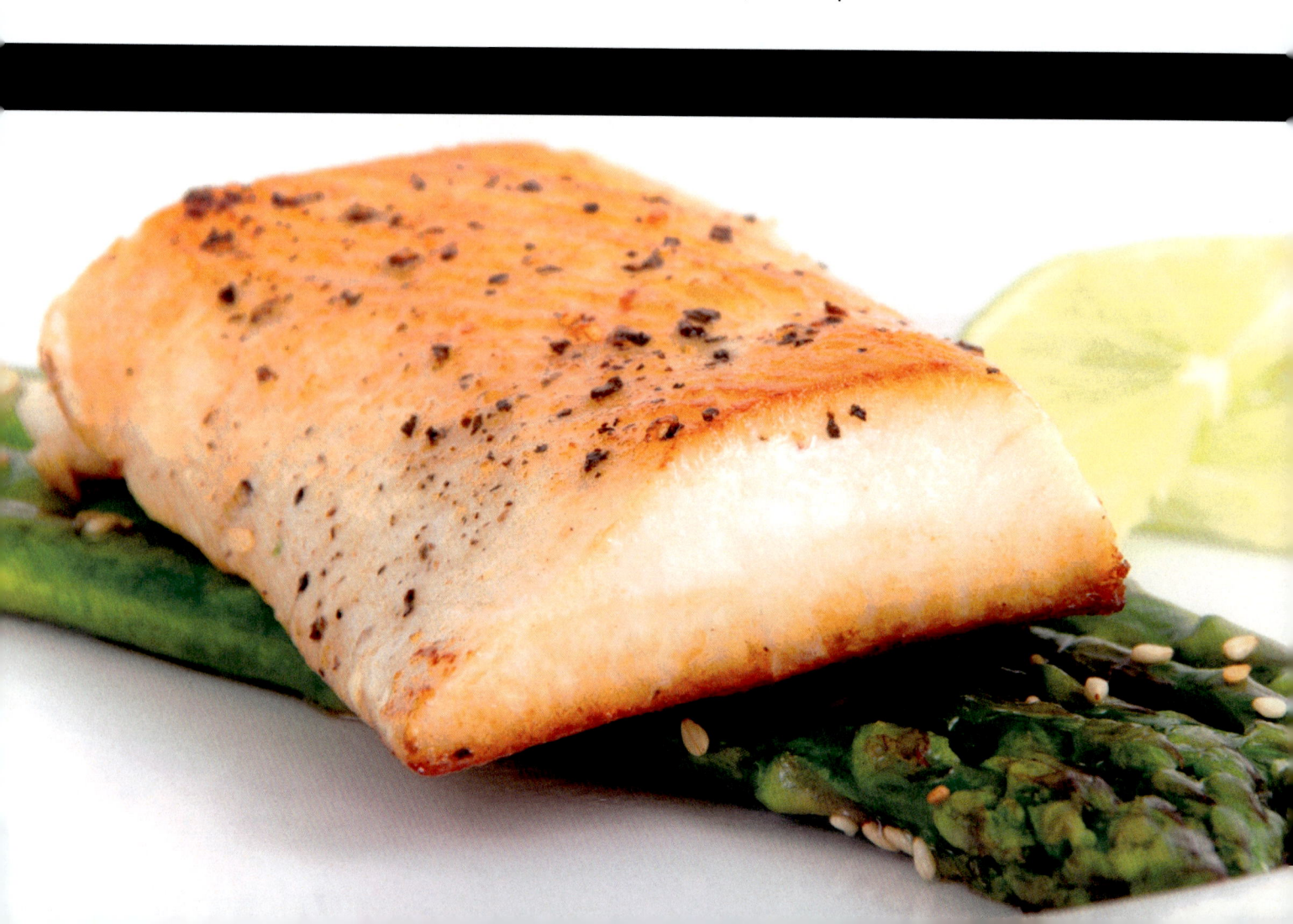

Directions

1. Preheat an outdoor grill for medium-high heat.

2. Place the wine and shallot in a saucepan over medium-high heat. Bring the mixture to a boil, then reduce the heat to medium-low and reduce the liquid down by about half, about 4 minutes. Remove from heat and set aside.

3. Place the Parmesan cheese, garlic, and walnuts into a food processor; process until finely chopped. Add melted coconut oil, cilantro, and 1/8 teaspoon black pepper; process until smooth. Remove the cilantro pesto from the food processor and set aside.

4. Place the red peppers into the food processor, pour in the wine reduction, and process until smooth. Pour the entire mixture back into the saucepan and bring to a boil over medium-high heat. Reduce the heat to medium and simmer the sauce for 4 minutes. Meanwhile, season both sides of the mahi mahi fillets with salt and pepper.

5. Cook the mahi mahi on the preheated grill until the fish is golden and flakes easily with a fork, about 4 minutes per side.

6. Whisk the butter, 1/8 teaspoon black pepper, and 1/4 teaspoon salt into the red pepper sauce until smooth. Spoon the red pepper sauce onto the bottom of the serving plate, arrange the fish on the sauce, and top with the cilantro pesto to serve.

Free Tools: SANESolution.com/Tools   Superfoods: store.SANESolution.com

Cajun Étouffée

Total Time: 1hr 10 min
Prep: 20 min
Cook: 50 min

8 Servings
1 Nutrient-Dense Protein Per Serving
1 Whole-Food Fat Per Serving

Ingredients

- 1/4 cup and 3 tablespoons extra virgin coconut oil
- 1/3 cup all-purpose flour
- 1-1/4 small green bell pepper, diced
- 1-1/4 medium onion, chopped
- 2-3/4 cloves garlic, minced
- 2-3/4 stalks celery, diced
- 2-3/4 fresh tomatoes, chopped
- 2 tablespoons and 2 teaspoons Louisiana-style hot sauce
- 1/2 teaspoon ground cayenne pepper (optional)
- 2 tablespoons and 2 teaspoons seafood seasoning
- 3/4 teaspoon ground black pepper
- 1-1/3 cups fish stock
- 1-1/4 pounds crawfish tails
- 1-1/4 pounds medium shrimp – peeled and deveined

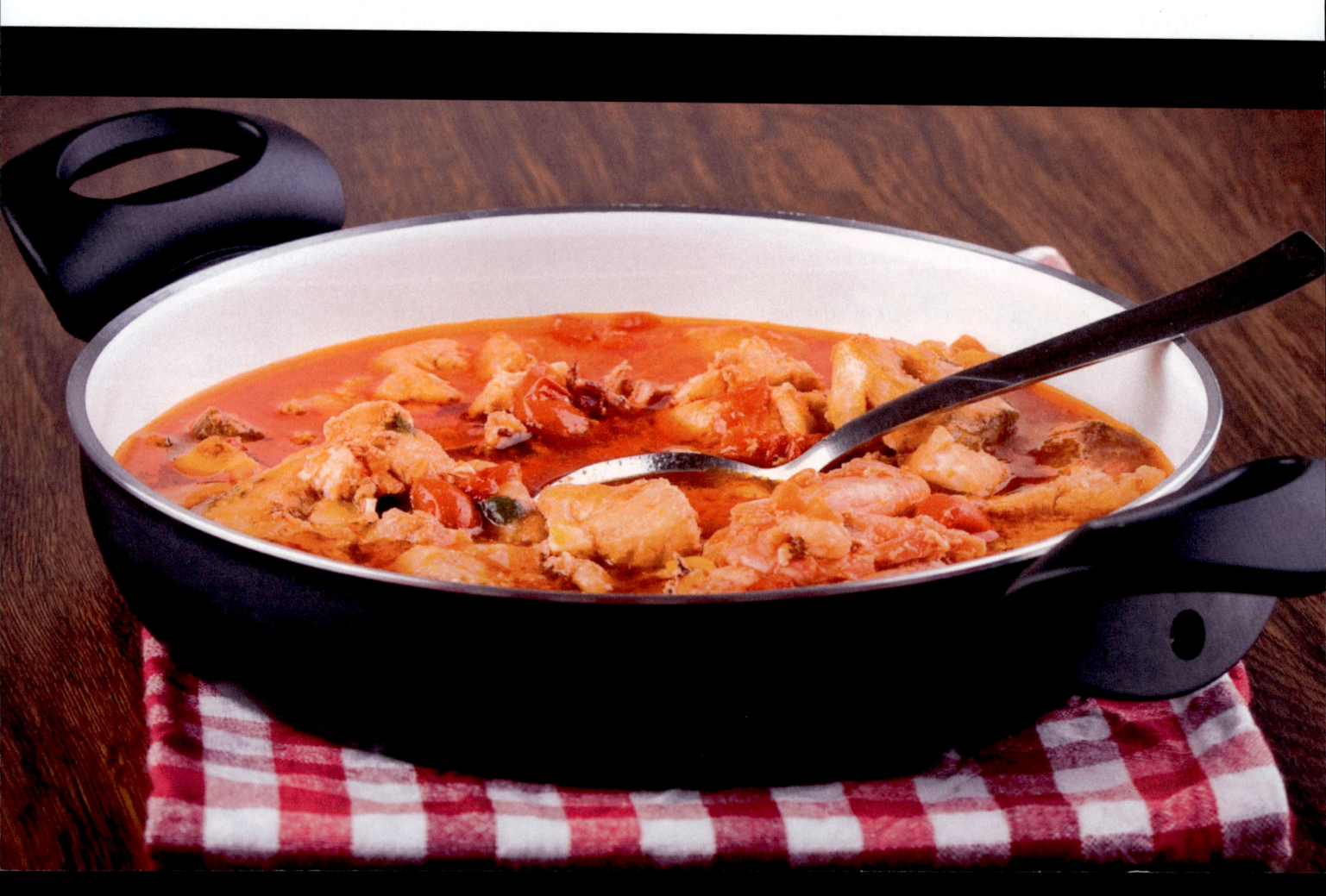

Directions

1. Heat the oil in a heavy skillet over medium heat. Gradually stir in flour, and stir constantly until the mixture turns 'peanut butter' brown or darker, at least 15 or 20 minutes. I use a large fork with the flat side to the bottom of the pan in a side to side motion. This is your base sauce or 'Roux'. It is very important to stir this constantly. If by chance the roux burns, discard and start over.

2. Once the roux is browned, add the onions, garlic, celery and bell pepper to the skillet, and saute for about 5 minutes to soften. Stir in the chopped tomatoes and fish stock, and season with the seafood seasoning. Reduce heat to low, and simmer for about 20 minutes, stirring occasionally.

3. Season the sauce with hot pepper sauce and cayenne pepper (if using), and add the crawfish and shrimp. Cook for about 10 minutes, or until the shrimp are opaque.

Seafood Stew

Total Time: 55 min
Prep: 10 min
Cook: 45 min

8 Servings
1 Nutrient-Dense Protein Per Serving
2 Whole-Food Fat Per Serving

Ingredients

- 1/3 cup and 2 tablespoons butter
- 1-1/4 onions, chopped
- 1-1/4 cloves garlic, minced
- 5/8 bunch fresh parsley, chopped
- 1-1/4 (14.5 ounce) cans stewed tomatoes
- 1-1/4 (14.5 ounce) cans chicken broth
- 1-1/4 bay leaves
- 1-3/4 teaspoons dried basil
- 1/4 teaspoon dried thyme
- 1/4 teaspoon dried oregano
- 1/2 cup and 2 tablespoons water
- 3/4 cup and 2 tablespoons and 2 teaspoons white wine
- 15 ounces large shrimp – peeled and deveined
- 15 ounces bay scallops
- 11 small clams
- 11 mussels, cleaned and debearded
- 3/4 cup and 2 tablespoons and 2 teaspoons crabmeat
- 15 ounces cod fillets, cubed

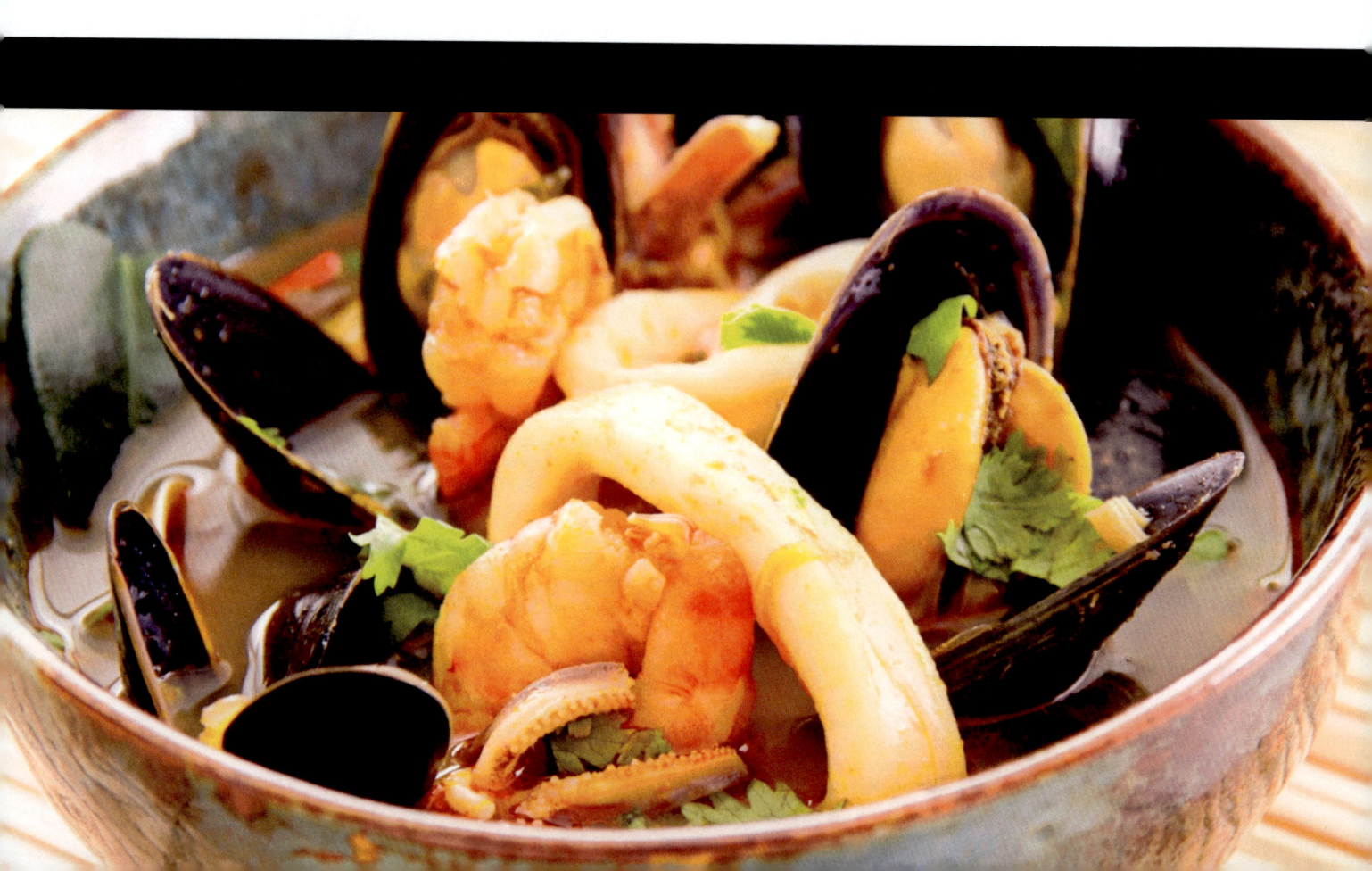

Directions

1. Over medium-low heat melt butter in a large stockpot, add onions, garlic and parsley. Cook slowly, stirring occasionally until onions are soft.

2. Add tomatoes to the pot (break them into chunks as you add them). Add chicken broth, bay leaves, basil, thyme, oregano, water and wine. Mix well. Cover and simmer 30 minutes.

3. Stir in the shrimp, scallops, clams, mussels and crabmeat. Stir in fish, if desired. Bring to boil. Lower heat, cover and simmer 5 to 7 minutes until clams open. Ladle soup into bowls and serve with warm, crusty bread!

SANE Free Tools: SANESolution.com/Tools Superfoods: store.SANESolution.com

Grilled Swordfish

Total Time: 22 min
Prep: 10 min
Cook: 12 min

8 Servings
2 Nutrient-Dense Protein Per Serving
1 Whole-Food Fat Per Serving

Ingredients

- 1/4 cup extra virgin coconut oil
- 1/2 cup lemon juice
- 1 tablespoon and 1 teaspoon Dijon mustard
- 1 tablespoon and 1 teaspoon finely chopped onion
- 1 teaspoon ground black pepper
- 2 teaspoons Cajun seasoning
- 2 teaspoons chopped fresh cilantro
- 2 pinches cayenne pepper, or to taste
- 8 (8 ounce) swordfish steaks

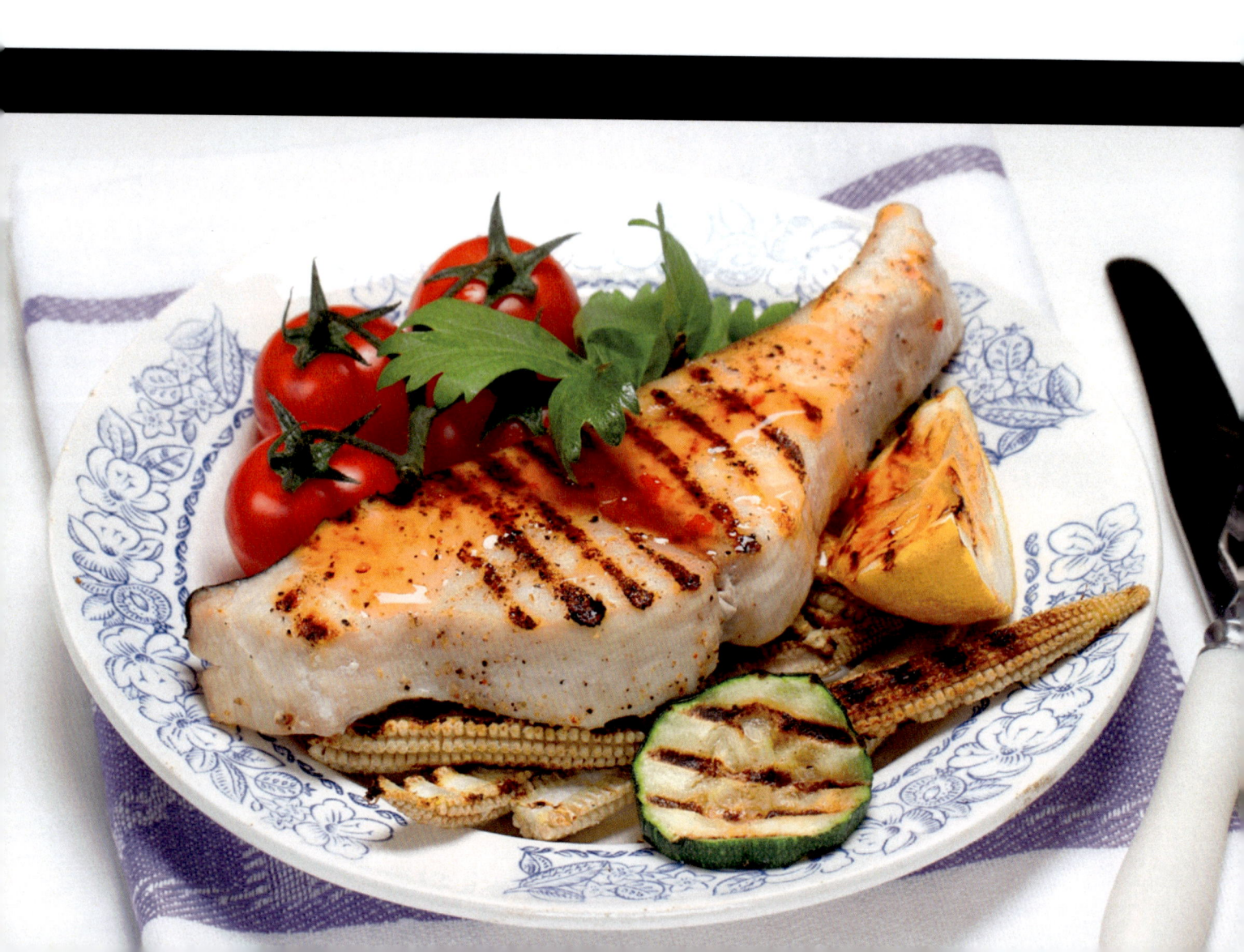

Directions

1. Combine extra virgin coconut oil, lemon juice, Dijon mustard, onion, black pepper, Cajun seasoning, cilantro, and cayenne pepper in a shallow glass baking dish. Add swordfish steaks, turning to coat with marinade. Cover and refrigerate for at least 30 minutes, turning occasionally.

2. Preheat an outdoor grill for high heat, and lightly oil the grate.

3. Grill swordfish steaks for 5 to 6 minutes on each side until the fish flakes easily with a fork.

So Much To Look Forward To...

You will learn much more about this as we start your personal weight-loss plan together in **your free half-day Masterclass** (reserve your seat at SANESeminar.com), but here are a few key reminders as you're getting started on your SANE journey.

SANE eating is a lifelong, enjoyable, sustainable, simple, and delicious way of eating. **It is not a repackaging of the unsustainable calorie counting diets that failed you.**

I know you understand this already—otherwise you wouldn't be here—but please keep in mind that since SANE isn't a calorie counting diet, you will not suffer through the same calorie counting tools and resources that failed you in the past. For example, **memorizing endless food lists and following unrealistic minute-by-minute meal plans aren't just a pain—they cannot work in the real world**, and they cannot work long term.

Life is crazy. Things happen. And heck, people have different tastes in food, so while minute-by-minute "eat exactly this right now no matter what" endless lists might make for good reality TV, if they worked in the real world, you would have already met your goals. **To get a different result (long-term fat loss and robust health), you MUST take a different approach.** That's what you will find here.

If you approach your new SANE life calmly, gradually, and with the next 30 years in mind rather than the next 30 days, **you will learn the underlying principles that enable you to make the SANE choices easily—forever**.

Think of your new approach as the difference between memorizing the sum of every possible combination of numbers versus learning the underlying principles of how addition works. Once you understand addition, lists and memorization aren't necessary as you know what to do with any combination of numbers—forever.

SANE   Free Tools: SANESolution.com/Tools   Superfoods: store.SANESolution.com

The same thing applies with food. Once you understand the new science of SANE eating, **you will know exactly what to eat (and what to avoid) everywhere you go—forever—without any lists** or any memorization.

This new approach changes everything and will forever free you from all the confusing and conflicting weight-loss information you've been told. So please allow me to congratulate you on coming to the life-changing realization that **to get different results than you've gotten in the past, you must take a different approach than you used in the past!**

The great news is that when you combine a calm, gradual, long-term, and progress vs. perfection mindset with your scientifically proven SANE tools, program, and coaching, you are **guaranteed to burn belly fat, boost energy, and enjoy an unstoppable sense of self-confidence!**

Your new SANE lifestyle has helped over 100,000 people in over 37 countries burn fat and boost health *long-term*....and it will do the same for you if you let it and trust it.

Thank you for taking the road less travelled...it will make all the difference!

SANEly and Gratefully,

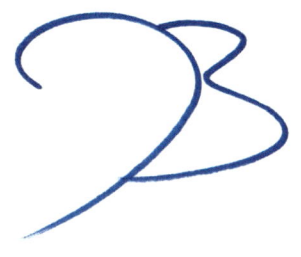

Jonathan Bailor | SANE Founder, NYTimes Bestselling Author, and soon...your personal weight-loss coach

P.S. Over the years I have found that our most successful members, the ones who have lost 60, 70, even 100 pounds... and kept it off... are the ones who start their personal weight-loss plan on...

our FREE half-day Masterclass. It's your best opportunity to fall in love with the SANE lifestyle, learn exactly how to start making the simple changes that lead to dramatic body transformations, and get introduced to your new SANE family. Be sure to reserve your spot at http://SANESeminar.com.

Please Don't Lose Your Seat at the FREE Masterclass Seminar!

Reserve your spot now so we can start your perfect personalized weight-loss plan. Space is limited and fills-up quickly. Reserve your spot now so you don't miss out!

Yes! I want to reserve my spot now at SANESeminar.com

About the Author: Jonathan Bailor is a New York Times bestselling author and internationally recognized natural weight loss expert who specializes in using modern science and technology to simplify health. Bailor has collaborated with top scientists for more than 10 years to analyze and apply over 1,300 studies. His work has been endorsed by top doctors and scientists from Harvard Medical School, Johns' Hopkins, The Mayo Clinic, The Cleveland Clinic, and UCLA.

Bailor is the founder of SANESolution.com and serves as the CEO for the wellness technology company Yopti®. He authored the New York Times and USA Today bestselling book *The Calorie Myth*, hosts a popular syndicated health radio show *The SANE Show*, and blogs on *The Huffington Post*. Additionally, Bailor has registered over 25 patents, spoken at Fortune 100 companies and TED conferences for over a decade, and served as a Senior Program Manager at Microsoft where he helped create Nike+ Kinect Training and XBox Fitness.

Improve Your Weight Loss, Energy, Mood, and Digestion In Just 17 Second A Day!

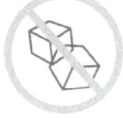

- 0g Sugar
- 100% Plant-Based
- Gluten Free
- No GMO's
- No Dairy
- No Soy

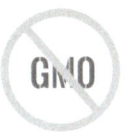

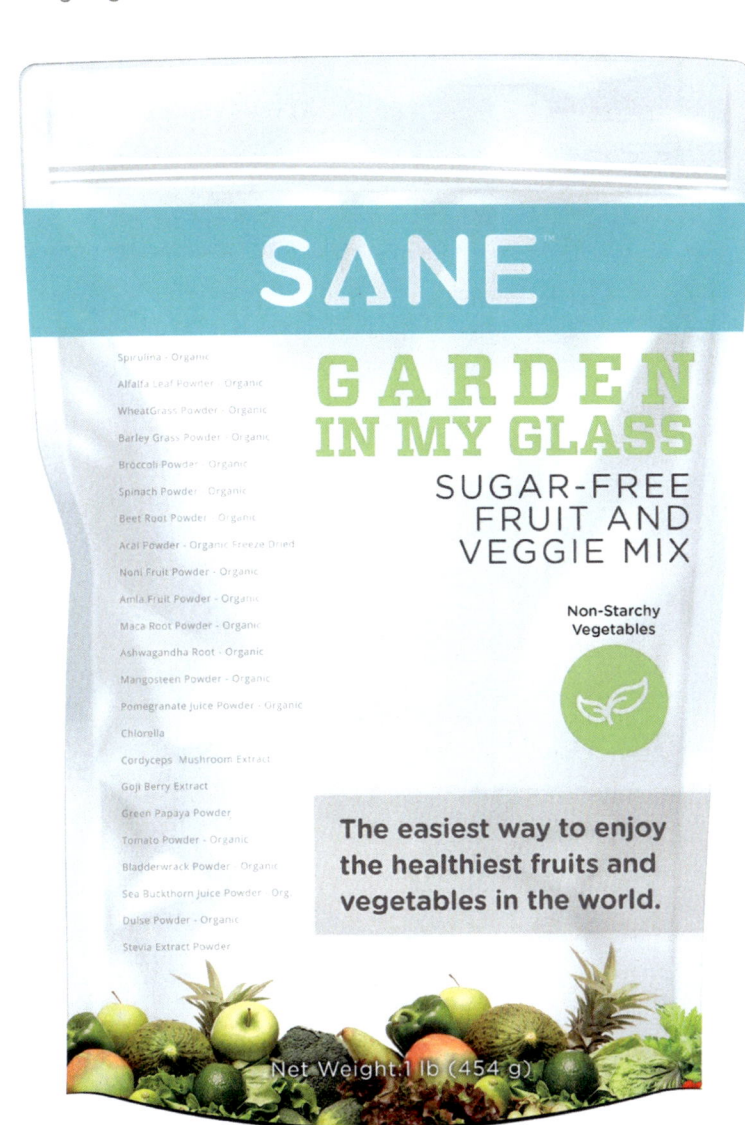

Introducing *Garden In My Glass*. The quickest, easiest, and most affordable way to get your family eating their fruits and veggies…and loving it!

When you order today you will also receive our wildly popular *'28 Days Of Green Smoothies'* recipe collection.

Plus, Get A Green Smoothie Recipe Book for FREE!

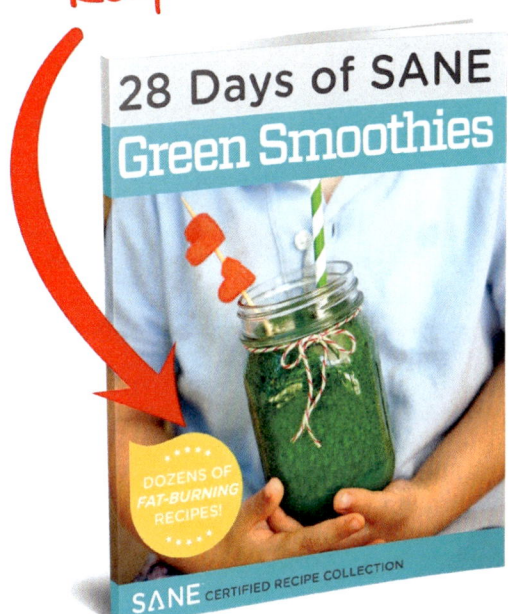

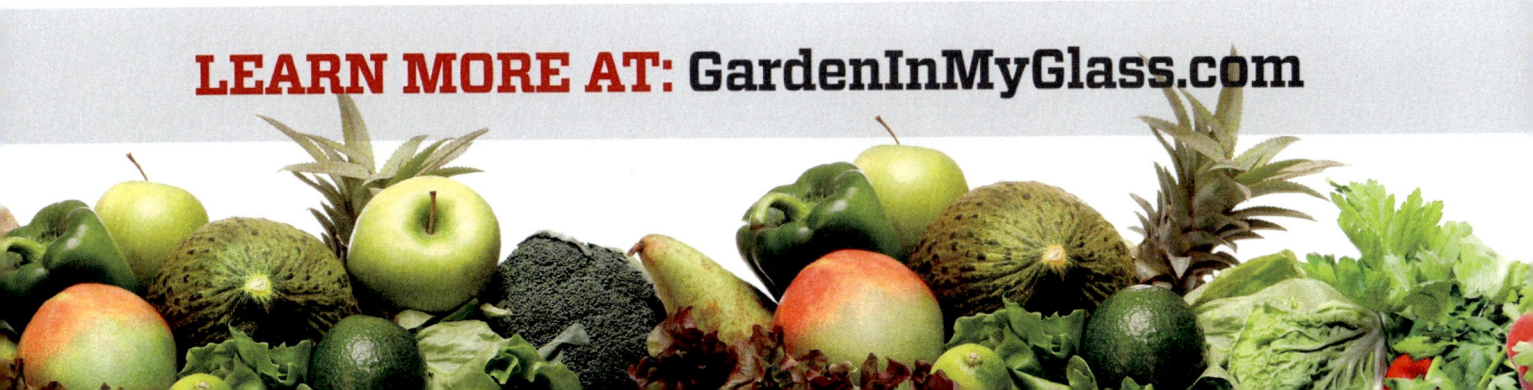

LEARN MORE AT: GardenInMyGlass.com

Get Everything You Need To Burn Fat and Prepare Delicious Meals at the SANE Store

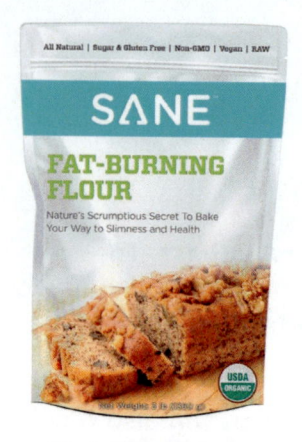

Fat-Burning Flour

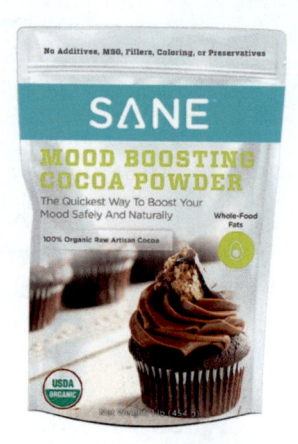

Mood-Boosting Chocolate Powder

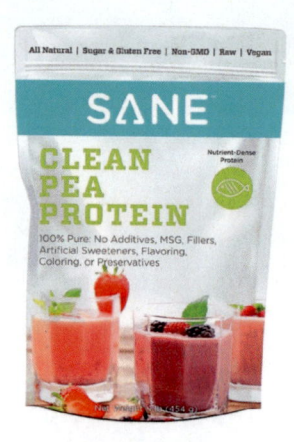

Clean Pea Protein

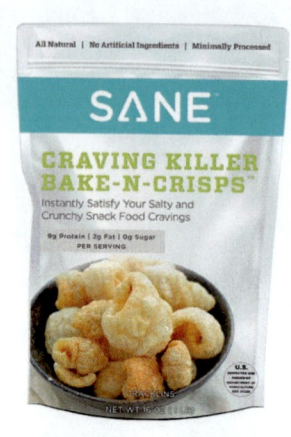

Craving Killer Bake-N-Crisps

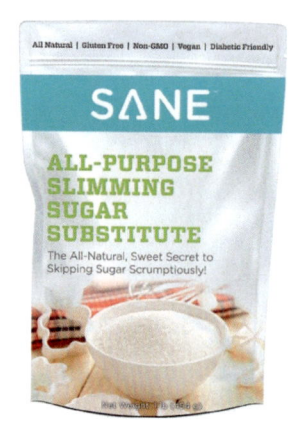

Slimming Sugar Substitute

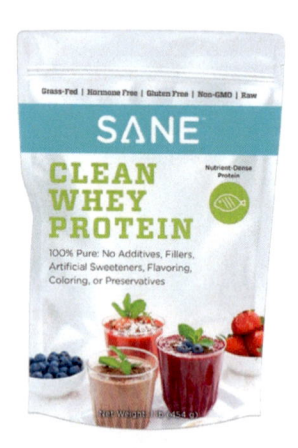

Clean Whey Protein

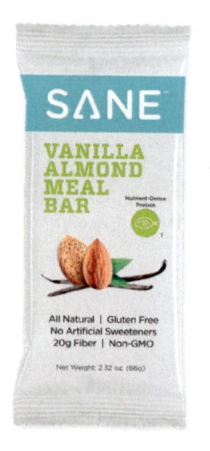

Vanilla Almond Meal Bars

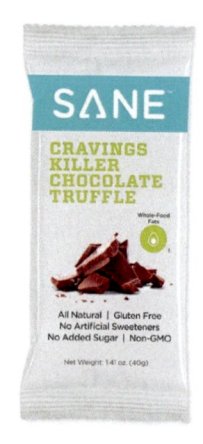

Craving Killer Chocolate Truffle

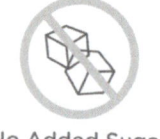

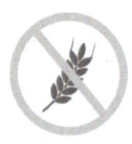

- No Added Sugar
- 100% Natural
- Gluten Free
- No GMO's
- No Dairy
- No Soy

SANE™

Find all of these EXCLUSIVE tools, plus over 100 other fat-burning SANE products to help you and your family look and feel your best!

Visit Today: Store.SANESolution.com

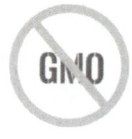

Made in the USA
Lexington, KY
20 February 2019